D0507448

ABOUT THE AUTHOR

Dr Kelly Neff is a social psychologist, author, professor, futurist and talk-radio personality who has electrified the transformational media world with her unique focus on the intersection of psychology, consciousness and human sexuality.

An academically trained research psychologist, she received her BA (2004) in Psychology *magna sum laude* and *Phi Beta Kappa* from Georgetown University and her MA (2006) and PhD (2010) in Social Psychology from Claremont Graduate University. She has spent nearly a decade as an associate professor of psychology, teaching both online and in-person Psychology of Human Sexuality courses at Saddleback College in California.

A millennial disrupter with a commitment to exploring the leading edge of psychology and technology, she wrote her first book, *Teaching Psychology Online* in 2013, and followed it up with articles on sex, consciousness, psychology and futurism that have been read and shared tens of millions of times across websites like *The Mind Unleashed, Wakeup World* and *MindBodyGreen*. Her hit show *Lucid Planet Radio* has attracted expert guests across the sciences, popular culture and esoteric traditions and has been streamed to hundreds of thousands of ears across the globe since it hit the airwaves in 2015.

Dr Kelly Neff's exuberant and engaging style has led to speaking engagements at both academic conferences and transformational events (like Sonic Bloom and Lucidity) across the US, demonstrating her ability to integrate her rigorous scientific training with her candid self-expression. *Sex Positive* (2020) epitomizes her desire to empower sexual freedom, inspire healing and improve people's relationships by fusing cutting-edge scientific findings with Eastern philosophies and her own deeply personal insights.

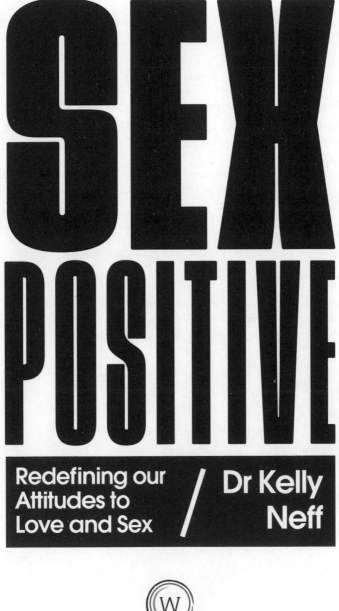

SEX POSITIVE

Redefining our Attitudes to Love and Sex / Dr Kelly Neff

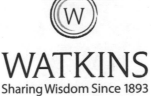

WATKINS

Sharing Wisdom Since 1893

This edition first published in the UK and USA 2020 by
Watkins, an imprint of Watkins Media Limited
Unit 11, Shepperton House
89–93 Shepperton Road
London
N1 3DF

enquiries@watkinspublishing.com
Design and typography copyright © Watkins Media Limited 2020
Text copyright © Kelly Neff 2020

Kelly Neff has asserted her right under the Copyright, Designs
and Patents Act 1988 to be identified as the author of this work.

All rights reserved.
No part of this book may be reproduced or utilized in any form
or by any means, electronic or mechanical,
without prior permission in writing from the Publishers.

1 3 5 7 9 10 8 6 4 2

Typeset by Lapiz
Printed and bound in the United Kingdom by TJ International

A CIP record for this book is available from the British Library

ISBN: 978-1-786782-95-3

www.watkinspublishing.com

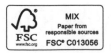

CONTENTS

INTRODUCTION

Cultivating Sex Positive Attitudes

I'm sure every generation feels this way, but my goodness, what an interesting and exciting time to be alive. Chaos is the only constant in a rapidly evolving world, and in our lives, we have surely experienced an unprecedented amount of change. Indeed, over the past three decades, human beings have witnessed a greater amount of technological development than in the previous 300 decades. We've seen more innovation happen at a faster pace than ever before, and we're just here trying to live our lives while we keep up! We have grown up, like no generation before us, with unparalleled access to every single piece of information out there, matched with an unlimited ability to connect to anyone in the world in the palms of our hands, 24/7/365. Our social and emotional development has unfolded enmeshed within social media and the worlds it creates, demanding that we maintain multiple identities and roles while offering us an audience for even our most mundane tasks.

It is hardly surprising then that *millennials* (the generation of people born between 1982 and 2000. Before you ask, yes! I'm an older millennial!) have already begun to redefine everything about love, sex and relationships. Disrupters of the status quo, we are developing increasingly positive, open-minded approaches to love and sex, shifting away from the negative, shameful connotations that have lingered for centuries. More than any generation before us, we are refusing to be categorized by gender stereotypes, embracing gender fluidity, reclaiming the female orgasm, pursuing non-monogamy, creating a whole new language for relational communication and opening ourselves up to incorporating many forms of technology in the bedroom. Our attitudes about love and sex are shifting dramatically and as the largest generation in human history, we are undoubtedly leaving the world an immensely different place from how we found it!

Growing up so intertwined with social media and screen time, it can sometimes feel challenging to express our unique identities and know what we really want out of relationships in this ever-changing world. These rapid changes over the course of only one generation can sometimes feel overwhelming and stressful. It can be easy to know what we don't want, but it can become a lot more challenging to figure out how to get what we *do* want. When it comes to what we want out of love, sex and relationships, the challenge to find our way could not be any more apparent. We want it all: We want to be happy! We want to love and accept ourselves, we deeply crave our independence, but we also want to be heard and understood. But how do we get there? How can we make sense of the major attitude swings happening in our generation? My hope is that this book can help illuminate the new narrative about love and sex, while offering tools for personal empowerment and insight into building healthy, sex positive relationships.

Rather than offering a purely academic or theoretical approach to our new psychologies about love and sex, I take a holistic approach to the topic that fuses my academic training with my personal story and experiences, highlighted within the context of our rapidly changing cultural climate. I believe that the best "self-help" offerings focus less on rigid prescriptive advice (as in, telling people what to do, which is not my style) and more on fluidly emphasizing the experience of deep introspection, nurturing critical thought, encouraging dialogue about complicated ideas and affording readers the means to make lasting changes to better their lives and relationships.

The Sex Positive Movement

Redefining sex and love as a constructive, harmonizing experience is a crucial part of how we move forward as a human collective. After so much struggle, anger and purging during the #MeToo movement over the past few years, the time has come for a new narrative that embraces sexual diversity, freedom and autonomy. One of the core concepts of this book is that we can flip the script by envisioning our bodies, desires and sexual experiences as naturally *positive* rather than inherently toxic or shameful. Of course, the universe is not all love and light and sometimes we do go through negative experiences. As we will learn, it is the way we cope with these struggles to become aware of our learned behaviour patterns and self-limiting beliefs that can reframe our sex positive futures. Out of this desire to rewrite the story of our lives in a way that mirrors our evolving attitudes, the sex positive movement was born.

The *sex positive movement* is a social, political and philosophical movement that promotes and embraces sexuality and sexual expression, with an emphasis on safe and consensual sex. Sex positive relationships are ones where partners support each other's choices and decisions without judgement, guilt or slut shaming. In a sex positive relationship, you can be whoever you want sexually, and do whatever you want sexually, without having to apologize for your sexual identity or expression, so long as you are not causing real harm to anyone else. In a sex positive relationship, you have permission to love your whole sexual body unconditionally, right now. Being sex positive can be best understood as a reaction to outdated misogynistic, patriarchal and religious structures that have sought to confine and control people's sexuality for far too long, and that crucially no longer serve us.

If you picked up this book, then being sex positive is probably either an attitude you already identify with, an attitude you are striving to cultivate or at least something you are curious about. If you are here because you desire a sex positive relationship, you have come to the right place. Or if you're reading this book because you don't know what else to do, but you know that you need relief from the pain and the hurting, you are still in the right place. It can be tough to stay positive when the world feels like such a toxic place, or when we feel disconnected and avoidant toward other people. Much of manifesting a sex positive relationship involves building your self-esteem so you are no longer afraid to assert your needs and desires, knowing that the right partner will honour them. Demand respect from yourself and the world and either you will get it, or you can walk away from anyone who does not value the person you are becoming.

The concept of the sex positive movement is one that I believe can benefit many people in all walks of life and relationships. It's not a movement solely for women, but one that can apply to all genders and lifestyles. Being sex positive is inherently inclusive, and this is the tone that I take in this book. Being sex positive is also something that applies to all types of past experiences, from people who are recovering from sexual abuse or trauma, to people who are searching for their voice and their sexual identity. It is important to remember that because of our social conditioning about sex we have all experienced some pain or hurt. I'm writing this book to let everyone out there know that you are not alone in this and that you deserve to understand and to heal.

Waking Up in the Time of #MeToo

It can be challenging to envision love and sex in a positive light when there is so much negativity out there in our media about intimacy and relationships. From 1 in 3 women across the world experiencing actual or attempted sexual assault, to transgender people being denied basic human rights, to the groundswell of #MeToo stories about people in positions of power using sex to take advantage of others, to men only being offered a narrow range of gender expressions that enforce anger and dominance while ridiculing sensitivity and gentleness, it seems that any chance of a narrative about healthy, happy sexuality has been twisted up and spat back out.

Yet perhaps we are missing an opportunity to find gratitude about how previously hidden issues regarding consent, harassment, gender, sexual orientation, intimate relationships and self-love have all been unprecedentedly brought to light in recent years, thanks to social media and our dialogues with our friends and loved ones. Just as many forms of psychological therapy involve a purging of repressed thoughts, feelings and memories, so too does our collective need to bring to the surface the misdeeds and the traumas that have happened so that we can build a new dialogue in order to move forward. As my psychology idol Carl Jung (who you will see quoted throughout this book) says, "one does not become enlightened by imagining figures of light, but by making the darkness conscious."[1] Over the past few years, we have begun to let our voices be heard about our traumas and our need to take our power back when it comes to our sexual identities, beliefs and desires. The outcry, rage and frustration had been pent up for far too long and it definitely needed to come out!

Instead of dwelling in the recesses of our pain, we must seek to blaze a path forward to rewrite and redefine the meaning of love and sex for our generation. We are disrupters by nature. But where do we even begin? Where is the frame of reference for building new personal and collective narratives about the true meaning of sexual empowerment?

First, we must remember that this crumbling patriarchal system as we know it is only one potential structure for societal organization. (The *patriarchy* refers to a social system or government where men hold primary power and predominant roles in political leadership, moral authority, social privilege and control of property.) For hundreds, maybe thousands of years, the true nature of our sexuality has been repressed by societal and religious institutions that have sought to control and manipulate the masses. We have not grown up in a world that encourages us to fully know and love ourselves as sexual beings. Many of us were raised to be fearful and shameful of sexuality, or conditioned by institutions, schools, corporations and the mass media to believe that only certain expressions of the sexual body, relationships and physical intimacy are appropriate. One could even go so far as to say that until very recently, our sexuality has been commoditized, and that our true nature as sexual beings suppressed.

But it has not always been this way. As you will learn in this book, for thousands of years before Western society even existed, Eastern and Indigenous Native traditions have long understood that the entire Universe operates as a sexual system, reflecting the balance of masculine and feminine energies that all people inherently possess regardless of their gender. Through achieving sexual harmony both within ourselves and in our relationships with intimate partners, we can unlock the keys to our health and wellness.

Consent is Sexy

In its rejection of toxic gender stereotypes, the #MeToo movement has sparked a crucial social dialogue about the importance of *consent*. Every person has a right to sexual autonomy, meaning that we maintain ownership over our bodies, and we have the right to say *no* to any sexual experience that makes us feel uncomfortable. We each possess a non-negotiable right to that *no* to be respected and heard. The *Tea Consent* video on You Tube offers must-watch viewing for those looking to clarify the true meaning of consent. Using the metaphor of offering someone a cup of tea (rather than offering sex), the video explains how just because you made someone tea does not mean you can force them to drink it. If someone says yes to tea but then decides they don't want to drink it, you don't make them drink it. If you make someone tea and they pass out before drinking it, you don't pour it down their throat while they are unconscious. What do you do for an unconscious person? You make sure they are *safe*.

This sounds pretty straightforward, right? A person who is intoxicated, unconscious or otherwise mentally incapacitated (or who is a child!) cannot legally give consent to engage in sexual behaviours (and they probably don't want any tea, either). When Stanford University student athlete Brock Turner only served three months in jail after being found guilty of sexually assaulting an unconscious woman on campus in 2015, the furious public outcry at his special treatment because of race and class privileges was akin to dumping gasoline on the flames of the #MeToo movement. While prosecutors recommended a six-year sentence for Turner, the judge who only sentenced him to six months (citing the potential "negative impact" of jail time on Turner's life) was recalled from active duty by California voters in 2018 (the first time this has happened in California since 1932). In a memorable groundswell of support, people collectively stood up against privileged men getting away with violating women's physical autonomy (perhaps Turner and Judge Aaron Persky should also have considered the "negative impact" of Turner's behaviour on the woman he attacked?). We should also remember how two other *males* at the college encountered Turner assaulting "Emily Doe" and restrained him until the authorities arrived, because the majority of men care about consent, too!

Tuner's case is only one of many where the perpetrator of sexual assault did not receive a just punishment, but it thrust the importance of consent into the national spotlight. The best sex, and the only type of sex in which we ought to participate as sex positive people, is *consensual sex*. I sometimes get laughed at when I say that consent is sexy, because some people think it ruins the moment when a partner needs to ask for permission to kiss you, or to touch your penis, or to have intercourse. But when you really think about it, does it get any sexier than someone who respects and cares enough about your safety to make sure you are completely comfortable? I don't think so. When in doubt, just ask. Can I touch you? Is this ok with you? This applies to people of all genders, not just the male in the relationship. If you're in a domestic partnership, a simple "do you want to have sex?" is a great way to start. And if your partner says no, then respect their wishes.

A number of issues have arisen in our dialogue about consent of late, including consent in the context of a marriage or domestic partnership, because contrary to fake old news, being married is not the same thing as giving consent to sex! While all 50 states have had *marital rape laws* on the books since 1993, they can be difficult to enforce because of loopholes. Consider the case of Jenny Teeson, who, while in the middle of a divorce in 2017, found a video of her husband sexually assaulting her with an object while she slept (she believes she was drugged when the video was taken). Teeson lives in Minnesota, where sex with someone who is physically helpless (as she was at the time) cannot be prosecuted as rape if the two people are married or domestic partners. Outraged that her husband was only charged with a misdemeanour and not a felony for the assault, Teeson led the charge at the state government level to change this law, and as of 2019, the bill to repeal this law (known as the "voluntary relationship defence") had passed the Minnesota House of Representatives (to the tune of Teeson receiving a standing ovation, no less). This example shows that while the #MeToo movement is helping to change public attitudes about consent, there are still many battles to be fought by brave individuals in this ongoing war over the respect for people's bodies and their choices.

A final thought on physical autonomy and consent: Consider the practice of male infant circumcision. While the scientific jury is still out on the extent of the trauma caused by the practice, it seems logical that removing the foreskin, one of the most sensitive parts of a boy's genitalia, *without his consent,* constitutes the sort of violation that we are better off without. When it comes to having autonomy over your body, for many men, it doesn't get much more sensitive than this! And who knows, maybe if we stop the practice of removing sensitive parts of boys' penises without their consent, they will grow up to be more respectful of other people's right to consent? (Just saying.)

This Book in Today's World

The ancient traditions remind us that humanity's sexual consciousness has been omnipresent for as long as we have been sexual beings. Yes, we may have lost our way, but the echoes of treating sex as an empowering experience has always been here, inside of each of us. However, the world we live in now is filled with challenges and pitfalls that are vastly different from the ones that any generation before us has faced.

The first part of the book, "Redefining Social Landscapes", examines how we have been programmed by "fake news" about who we are, and how we are rejecting many of these socially conditioned attitudes in favour of a more fluid and inclusive approach. We will also explore the crucial role of technology, specifically the "technosexual revolution", in completely redefining our attitudes about sexual intimacy, what turns us on, and what love and sex really mean.

The second part of the book, "Redefining Ourselves", delves deeper into how the nature of our identities and personal feelings about ourselves as sexual beings has begun to shift. We will explore evolving attitudes about sexuality as a "spiritual" experience, as well as how we can reclaim and redefine the very nature of orgasm. Then, we will focus on how to cope with the transformation in our attitudes and identities through the lens of our inner landscapes, including acknowledging our traumas, recognizing programmed beliefs, practising self-love, finding forgiveness and cultivating a state of flow. All of this is essential *before* we begin to involve ourselves in building sex positive relationships.

Finally, in part three of the book, "Redefining Our Relationships", we explore what we really want in relationships, and how to find the "right" partner for a sex positive intimate connection, featuring theories from psychology as well as from the esoteric traditions. We will explore the evolution of fluid relationship configurations, particularly non-monogamy, as well as the new styles of relationship communication our generation has developed in tandem with social media. Finally, we explore some of the pitfalls of online dating communication, as well as solutions to help you build a sex positive relationship in the face of so much chaos and confusion.

My Journey

A huge part of my inspiration to write this book comes from my personal journey recovering from sexual body trauma and connecting to my sex positive attitudes – but a few caveats before I begin.

First and most importantly, I will never lose faith in people's abilities to reinvent themselves, even in the face of scarring challenges and uncertainty. Maybe it is only through a trauma that we can learn our strengths and process the lessons we need to become happier, more well-adjusted people. But that doesn't make it any easier when we are suffering, grieving and purging through the pain of what has happened to us. Second, I am and will always be an optimist, based on my belief that we can always find another chance, a way to change, or a path to reinvention. And third, I want you to know my story so that you can see my biases and my perspective.

When it comes to the scientific method, as researchers we are encouraged to remain impartial and not put our biases or emotions into our work. But when it comes to the topic of sex and relationships, how can anyone really remain as such? Being impartial is not my aim in writing this book. My goal is to be real, and to show you myself in hopes that the reflection will help you to illuminate yourself. I am fallible, I have made many of my own mistakes, and I do not want you to believe that I have all of the answers. I might have advanced degrees and many years working with people in this field, but what makes me able and qualified to write this book is not my academic training, but my humanity and my love for people and desire to help them heal and build happy lives.

With that said, let me tell you my story. First of all, like many people, I have always liked sex and I have been sexually active for as long as I can remember. I remember experimenting when I was kid. I remember how much I enjoyed myself the first time I gave a guy oral sex. Turns out, it was a terrible idea to tell most of my friends in my class about it. Within a few hours, this news circulated the school and I became one of the "class sluts". I still couldn't exactly understand why what I did was wrong, or how the way that I was treated should be any different from the way the same guy was being treated for getting oral sex in the first place.

After that, something started to shift inside of me. Experiencing the sexual double standard first-hand when I was at such an awkward age socially, I began to feel enraged inside. Why should women be afraid of sex and shamed for it, while men were applauded for it? I felt incredibly angry inside that I couldn't express myself the way I wanted to as a sexual being without being subjected to torrents of abuse and ridicule. I may have been young, but I felt mature enough to demand my sexual autonomy! Now, this was in the late 1990s, and I wonder if things would have been very different today, for better or, probably, for worse. Something started happening around this time though, which is that my periods became extremely and brutally heavy.

Immensely frustrated by my experiences in adolescence, as a young adult I tried to hide my sexuality. After years of fighting to be accepted and not judged for being a sexually autonomous being, I started to feel like maybe there was something wrong with me after all. I settled into a long-term relationship, I kept the fact that I was bisexual to myself, and I barely had sex at all. And in what was perhaps not a coincidence, after years of physical torment with my periods, I had to seek medical help. I was told that I had polyps, cysts and uterine fibroids and during my mid-to-late 20s I underwent four separate surgeries to have the growths removed, all unsuccessful. During this time, I was also in graduate school and teaching human sexuality, pushed to the absolute brink of exhaustion and pain from the constant bleeding – sex seemed like a distant memory.

By the time I was 31, I was in a new relationship with a man who encouraged me to express my sexuality. I think he could understand and feel the pain that I had been in, believing it might help my condition if I started to connect with that part of myself again. He also taught me Reiki, which is a form of energy healing channelled through the healer's hands, and he would frequently use this healing technique on me when my pain became unbearable.

That June, the bleeding started one morning and did not stop. I thought I was probably going to die. It was 3 am but my partner scooped me up and drove me to the emergency room. They took a blood test and my blood haemoglobin was a 4.0, when it should be over 12.0. They told me I could have had a stroke at any time and were shocked that I was walking. My uterus had taken all of the blood in my body and bled nearly all of it out.

I found myself in triage with the worried-looking doctors sticking needles in my arms and asking if I had ever had a blood transfusion. I begged them for something to assuage the anxiety building up inside of me. They were going to give me a placebo to try to calm me down so that I would accept the blood transfusion. When the doctor came back in, he put an injection into my IV line and told me it was alprazolam (but it was really saline). Do you know what happened? I calmed down and instantly relaxed. I will never forget this moment because it showed me first-hand the incredible power of the mind over the body.

During the days that followed when I was in the ICU fighting for my life, I had a series of experiences that I can only explain as near-death hallucinations or out-of-body experiences. Later one night when things were very touch and go, I left my body and found myself in a hallucination on the ethereal plane talking to none other than Krishna, the holy Hindu deity of life, which even at the time seemed odd because I didn't believe in the Hindu gods at all.

When it finally came to surgery day, I was still fairly anaemic. The surgery ended up taking several hours longer than planned, because instead of two tumours in my uterus they found over two thousand. They were forced to perform an emergency hysterectomy (meaning that they had to remove the entire uterus) and I was told later it was the size of a seven-month pregnancy! While I felt very grateful to have survived, I remained in a complete emotional mess for months after as I tried to integrate and process this traumatic experience. I don't really remember much from this time except a state of deep shock that all of this had happened. I never got an explanation for why my uterus was so messed up, nothing hormonal, or genetic, or illness based or anything. There was no explanation! This tormented me for a long time until I realized that the answer was right in front of me all along: What if I was somehow responsible for creating this monster? What if by repressing my sexual energy and internalizing the guilt and shame directed to me for so long, I somehow made myself extremely sick? If my mind has enough power to tell the body what to do when it comes to the placebo, doesn't this mean my mind has more power over my body than I ever gave it credit for?

Naturally, the course of my life began to shift paths. I found myself moving further away from conventional science and closer to studying energy, consciousness and frequencies as a way to make sense of our world. Looking back, I believe that part of the mission has been connecting to this deeper knowledge and passing it on to help others heal.

If we want to love our sexual bodies and repair our broken psychologies about sex, maybe we must connect to our higher levels of consciousness that deal in energy, frequency and vibration. I know that this place is real to me because I have experienced it first-hand. While I will never be able to get my uterus back, and I cannot prove any of this, I can move forward, almost like I have been strangely reborn into a new timeline with a new life. Now, there is no more pain. I am free to live, to work and to take chances without slowly dying one day at a time. My gratitude for this path, and how it put my life back together so that I could learn this lesson, is why I will never give up on people no matter how messed up they might seem in any given moment. And it is why I believe that everyone should have the opportunity to embrace sex positive attitudes. We are all navigating the shift together. If I can make it through my sexual body trauma, I firmly believe that you can make it through anything, too.

If you want to be part of the sex positive movement, it doesn't matter what your gender is, or your sexual orientation, or if you are a survivor of sexual trauma or not. What matters is that you are willing to accept people's sexualities as long as they are consenting and not causing harm to anyone else. As we will learn, holding onto toxic anger, directed at ourselves or at anyone who inflicted pain upon us, will hinder our ability to heal. We have to rise above our pain and to give everyone the chance to either reinvent themselves or assert their respect for sexual autonomy before we refuse to include them in the new story about sex. This is the true path to revolution, with nobody left behind. Throughout this journey, please keep in mind the ways that your attitudes and feelings will continue to evolve. And you should probably strap yourself in, because the revolution has already begun! It is time explore how we are rewriting the story of sex and love, beginning with our changing social landscapes.

PART ONE
REDEFINING SOCIAL LANDSCAPES

CHAPTER I
FAKE NEWS

Ah, *fake news*. I'm pretty sure this might have been the most popular new phrase of the past few years! It seems rather appropriate that a discussion of redefining *anything* important about our attitudes would naturally begin with a deconstruction of the fake news about who we are – the fake news we have received through socialization. While cries of "fake news" in our sociopolitical climate are usually a way of mudslinging the lack of fact-checking between politicians and journalists, when it comes to sex, love and relationships, our version of "fake news" involves the lies we have been told about who we are as sexual beings. Almost everything we have been taught about our gender norms, our sexual desires, our bodies and so on reflects a culturally conditioned story rooted less in fact than in fiction.

For centuries, our culture has dictated the range of behaviours that are socially acceptable for us. We are taught from birth how to be male or female, often becoming deeply entrenched in the behaviours, roles and feelings associated with our assigned genders. We learn what we can and can't do or say when it comes to our sexuality. Many of us come of age under a veil of religious shame and come to believe that sex is somehow shameful or bad. We grow up in a world with massive sexual double standards for men (players and studs) versus women (virgins or sluts). We are also taught about acceptable and unacceptable body types and are conditioned by the mass media to believe that only some are attractive. Much of what we think we *know* about our sexual selves feels true because we have believed it for so long.

And yet, droves of us are fighting back against this programmed fake news about sex, reclaiming our identities and demanding a total rewrite of the story, replacing it with one that is more coherent with our desires for fluidity and freedom. The transformation we are living through right now feels so extreme that the world we are crafting might look less like a revision of the story and more like burning the entire book and starting again. It is an incredibly exciting time to be alive when it comes to new ideas about masculinity and femininity (if those terms still have any meaning, that is). We are disrupting the narrative about love, sex and gender that has dominated human identities for centuries. What will replace them? What will the future of love and sex look like if we stay on our current course?

Wise people say that to understand the future, we must first understand the past. I find this to be a useful notion when we are thinking about redefining love and sex. We need to figure out exactly how we got to this unique place where we suddenly find it not only important but 100 per cent necessary to craft a new story about our sexual identities. What happened to us that stripped away our power to express ourselves outside of the norm? What can we learn from the past that will help us build a future that is more in line with our core values?

The Psychology of Social Conditioning

Social conditioning refers to the psychological process of training individuals in a society to respond and behave in a manner that is generally approved by the society and its relevant peer groups. Going back to my story in the introduction, a teenage girl telling everyone how much she liked sex was met with shame and ridicule from my peers, who were conditioning me to stick to the social norm that teenage girls aren't supposed to like sex. I was punished for deviating from a relatively oppressive social norm, but did my classmates even know they were doing this?

Probably not. I doubt that someone literally said, "Hey, she stepped out of line! Shame her so she conforms to the social norms!" Rather, they were acting unconsciously based on what they had been taught, that violating the commonly held rules about sexuality comes with enforceable consequences.

If you're like me, you're probably reading this and thinking, "*Screw that*! I am who I am, and I make choices based on my feelings, not what anyone has ever told me to do." And I say, good for you. But nobody is immune to social conditioning. Even if you grew up with not one human around and you were raised by wolves in the forest, you'd probably end up socially conditioned by the wolves. Humans do not exist in a cultural vacuum: We encounter thousands of messages every day from institutions, media and advertising, and possibly even more nowadays than ever before because we often access multiple screens simultaneously. Perhaps the images that we are fed repeatedly do influence us unconsciously even when we consciously reject them.

Our culture affects us through a process known as *socialization*, which is best described as the internalization of commonly accepted values, beliefs and norms. The nature versus nurture debate in psychology is this: Do our intrinsic, dispositional traits (*nature*) make us who we are, does our environment including our families, schools, religious institutions and media determine who we become (*nurture*)? The debate rages on but I believe that both socialization and nature interact; one doesn't dominate over the other. Think about your own life story: Have you always felt a "certain way" about your gender identity or have you been influenced by the people around you? What about your sexuality: Which has been more pervasive, your own desires or those of the people and institutions in your environment?

The Fake News Narrative on Gender

Before you say that socialization hasn't affected your attitudes about love and sex, consider what we have been taught about gender. *Gender* refers to the attitudes, feelings and behaviours that a given culture associates with a person's biological sex. Embedded in gender is a set of socially constructed *gender roles* teaching us which activities and attributes our society deems appropriate for men and women. We've been conditioned to accept the legitimacy of these roles, which can lead to the perpetuation of gender stereotypes (a *stereotype* is a widely accepted judgement or bias about a person or group that is usually oversimplified and can be inaccurate).

Stereotypes about gender in particular can cause unfair and unequal treatment of an individual because of their gender. This is called *sexism* and although we traditionally associate it with women, sexism is gender blind because it can happen to men and to transgender people, too. Gender stereotypes play out across a variety of different dimensions including *personality traits* (for example, women are expected to be emotional whereas men are expected to be aggressive), *domestic behaviours* (women are expected to cook and clean while men repair the house), *occupations* (assuming nurses and teachers are female while engineers and pilots are male) and *physical appearance* (women are expected to be thin and glamorous whereas men are expected to be big and strong). Yes, men and women have different levels of the sex hormones (oestrogen, testosterone) and varied body compositions. And yes, some of these stereotypes might be in sync with an underlying reality for some people. Problems arise when we are conditioned to believe that these roles are the *only* acceptable options, or when we make assumptions about other people based solely on these stereotypes.

In a rather sensationalist 2017 headline, *USA Today* claimed that "Gender Stereotypes Are Destroying Girls and They're Killing Boys."[2] This article was based on findings published in the *Journal of Adolescent Health* (2017) showing how the gender stereotypes internalized in adolescence can lead to damaging consequences into adulthood. Data analyses from 15 countries across five continents from the *Global Early Adolescent Study* exposed the single most damaging gender stereotype: The *hegemonic myth* that once they hit puberty, girls become vulnerable while boys become independent.[3] This attitude was conditioned by seemingly everyone, from schools, to parents, to the media – and even by peers.

In the study, the notion that girls require protection once they hit puberty became internalized by both genders as early as age ten, creating a narrative of pubertal girls as victims and pubertal boys as sexual predators. Wrapped up in the hegemonic myth were several related stereotypes such as the belief that girls embody sexuality and must therefore avoid dressing in certain ways or engaging in certain behaviours that could trigger boys' and men's aggressive and exploitative tendencies. Girls came to internalize these norms to a greater extent than boys in some settings. Sound familiar? Think about the rape myths still being propagated worldwide that wearing sexy clothes or attracting male attention means that a woman is somehow to blame for being assaulted by a man. If adolescent boys and girls are being socialized to believe this myth, how can we expect them to think any differently as adults?

Due to the pervasiveness of these gender stereotypes, girls in the study found their mobility significantly more limited than that of the boys as they were taught to "cover up and don't go out". The myth of boys as troublemakers and aggressors was equally prevalent, which evokes a chicken versus egg debate about whether men are naturally aggressive, or whether they are acting in socially conditioned ways. Adolescent girls also feared sanctions ranging from punishment, sexual rumour, social isolation and innuendo for spending time with the same boys they played with as children. Most adolescents in the study were saddened by the situation but were acutely aware of consequences levelled toward their peers who did not conform to these stereotypes, with analyses showing that boys were even less tolerant than girls of their same gender peers who did not conform to their appropriate gender roles.

The majority of research on adolescent gender stereotypes alludes to devastating consequences for girls who are taught that they are weak, as well as for boys who are taught that they are troublesome predators. In the study, adherence to these gender stereotypes in adolescent girls was linked to depression, leaving school early and exposure to violence later in life. Boys were also not as unscathed from these myths as popular opinion might like to suggest: In fact, boys who internalized the hegemonic myth were more likely to engage in and become victims of physical violence and were more prone to substance abuse and suicide.[4]

These findings show how harmful it can be when we label people and place expectations upon them just because of their gender. Some readers might try to argue that these global stereotypes do not necessarily apply to life in the US, or the UK or other Western countries. Still, we often witness elements of the hegemonic myth of vulnerable girls and aggressive boys across Westernized society. Consider multiple news headlines of girls being sent home from school for dressing "too promiscuously", often for wearing a tank top and/or a short skirt. In 2019, a Kentucky teenager made the headlines after being sent home from school for wearing a pair of short overalls (dungarees) that were not in any way revealing, at least in my opinion. Courtney Robertson, 15, said she was "humiliated" and "disgusted" after her teacher said she "acted like she was a whore". The fallout? The teen says, "I genuinely feel like sh*t now. I absolutely hate my body image."[5] Do boys ever experience the same extreme dissection and critique of their appearance or clothing choice? Has a boy ever been sent home from school for wearing "revealing" clothing? Or what about girls being told that they cannot play certain sports like wrestling or football, because they might get hurt or be leered at by the boys?

No, She's Not Asking for It!

When it comes to sex, the *double standard* remains one of the most prevalent fake old news stereotypes, alluding to the idea that a woman who enjoys sex is a *slut* whereas a man who does the same should be deemed a *stud* or a *player*. (Based on my past experiences, I have reclaimed slut as a term of endearment, that

YES, I am a woman and YES, I enjoy sex! If that makes me a slut, then I embrace it openly! I have a clitoris and a G spot for a reason, honey!)

Embodied in this double standard is the idea that a woman who dresses sexily or provocatively deserves to be harassed or assaulted, whereas one who dresses conservatively is a prude deserving of ridicule or attempts to unlock her sexuality. The problem with this stereotype is that either way, people lose when they are objectified by the way they look. The idea that a woman dressed provocatively in a skirt or a low-cut top somehow deserves assault or unwarranted male sexual attention remains one of the most commonly perpetuated rape myths. *No, she's not asking for it!* People can dress however they want regardless of gender – and while others may choose to make judgements, the simple truth is that what people wear does not necessarily reflect their sexuality. Women are allowed to wear whatever they choose. So are men. So are trans people. Clothing choice *never* equals consent.

The best way to start deprogramming yourself regarding gender stereotypes is to become aware of how this prescriptive way of teaching may have affected your attitudes and your identity. If you are a woman, were you ever taught that you were too vulnerable to go out by yourself? Do you still feel that way? If you are a man, were you taught to believe that you were an aggressive person solely because of your gender? If you are transgender or gender fluid, have you felt conflicted about how to manifest your masculine, feminine or gender neutral attributes? How might these stereotypes still affect your identity as an adult?

Gender stereotypes reinforce a broken binary opposition that pits women and their perceived weaknesses versus men and their supposed aggression. The hegemonic myth reflects narrow and inaccurate ways of looking at the world and categorizing people from a limiting biological standard. The very fact that some men continue to use feminized words like "pussy" or "mangina" to insult one another for not being strong or virile enough helps to reinforce this point. People say "grow some balls!" which seems hilarious and ironic because we all know that the testicles are some of the most sensitive organs in the whole body! Who could forget the saying, "If you want to be tough, grow a vagina! Those things can take a pounding."

As our culture continues to evolve, we will continue to fight against fake old news, which is a remnant of Victorian-era beliefs about sexuality that still infest our social worlds today. The idea that women should be quiet and reserved whereas men should be loud and boisterous; the notion that women should be emotional whereas men should be stoic; the mere concept that women need to protect themselves from men's violent sexual urges and should never actually enjoy sex – all of this is fake old news from a not so distant past where women did not have the right to vote, weren't allowed to hold down jobs or leave their houses without an escort and were expected to wear corsets so tight they could barely breathe. Oh, and if they were empowered or if they enjoyed sex in any way, women were subjected to a wide range of consequences ranging from being burnt at the stake as a witch to being diagnosed as a "nympho" or "hysterical" and having their ovaries brutally removed.

It has been about 100 years since these myths were considered irrefutable, and while today women have many more rights, some parts of society are taking longer to catch up. According to the Institute for Women's Policy Research, in 2017 women in America still earned an average of 20 per cent less for doing the exact same job as a man, and the amount is even lower for women of colour.[6] Women are not offered standard paid maternity leave in the US, while many other countries offer paid leave to both mothers and fathers. Yet, more than any other generation before us, we are the most supportive of shared housework and household chores. The share of millennial women with bachelor's degrees even now exceeds the number of millennial men with bachelor's degrees.[7]

Given young women's educational attainments and career goals (34 per cent of millennial women aspire to be the boss at work while only 24 per cent of millennial men do), why are they earning less than their male peers? Perhaps we can thank fake old news for helping to build the glass ceiling many women hope to shatter.

Are you angry about the idea of our future generations internalizing more of these hegemonic, limiting gender stereotypes? You have a right to be. We are already leading by example by supporting people who reject gender stereotypes when they emerge in our daily lives. Gender equality is long overdue, from ending the gender pay gap, to giving both men and women paid maternity leave, to female lead characters who don't need a man to rescue their vulnerable selves (Hello, *Captain Marvel!*), to seeing body positive adverts that feature a variety of body types for men, women and trans people. We are starting to make this the legacy we leave behind.

Fake News about Sexual Relationships

In terms of sexual relationships, another common stereotype is that only men want one-night stands whereas women want romance, marriage and long-term commitments. Once again, fake old news is being perpetuated by thousands of movies and books from the 20th century and earlier. In reality, there are plenty of women out there who want one-night stands, and plenty of men who want commitment. We are all human beings: We all want different things and that is alright! Still, it is easy to become frustrated with self-help books and magazine advice columns which unfairly assume that all women want committed relationships while all men just want to "use them" for sex. This kind of narrow-minded approach does not help anyone and just seeks to further pit masculinity and femininity in opposition to one another. As we will learn later in the book, sexual scripts that emphasize orgasm as the goal of sex, or that a vaginal orgasm is somehow "superior" to a clitoral orgasm, or that women do not have strong sex drives, are starting to take on much less meaning. Our sexual scripts are rapidly evolving, and many of these stereotypes and dated beliefs simply no longer apply.

Sexualized Parts of the Body

Social conditioning has also taught us about the acceptable and unacceptable versions of the body, based mostly upon representations of the sexual body and genitalia in popular culture. Thanks to the massive viewership of pornographic magazines, movies and websites (the impact of which we will discuss in chapter 3) typically only a narrow range of sexual bodies and genitals remains externally visible in our culture. Men with muscles and large, thick penises and women with vaginas that typically have almost no protruding labia have become the norm. Could this be why the practice of labiaplasty in America (a cosmetic surgery procedure to reduce the size of the labia) has increased at a rate of nearly 40 per cent per year?[8]

Please remember that the sexual body comes in so many shapes and sizes and is just as diverse as the rest of human sexuality. Quodoushka Native American teachings highlight "nine types of vaginas" and "nine types of penises" that have been passed down through their sexual knowledge traditions. They postulate that the size and shape of a person's genitals will determine the type of pleasure that they receive from different kinds of sexual experiences. It is a common misconception that everyone out there finds the genitals they see in porn to be the most attractive or the only attractive option. Just because your body does not look like what you see elsewhere does not mean that your genitals are not normal. No matter how they look, there is a huge diversity in human genitalia and yours are just fine.

Another myth about sexual bodies surrounds the need to censor women's nipples. The "free the nipple" campaign has sparked tons of controversy on social media, where images of women's nipples are generally censored or deemed "obscene" – but not men's nipples. Artistic images celebrating and empowering the female body are consistently still taken down due to "community standards" on Facebook and Instagram, much to my total outrage. Why is a topless woman somehow more upsetting or provocative than a topless man? This philosophy treats the natural female body as though it is a sex object to be lusted after, invoking the threat of the hegemonic myth that men are predators and cannot control themselves. Not to mention the fact that in most places in America, women cannot publicly display their nipples for fear of violating obscenity laws, but nearly every 7-11 or corner store sells multiple magazines featuring topless women. This teaches us a message that it is ok (and legal) to sell women's breasts in America, but not ok (nor legal) to wear women's breasts in America. WTF?

Other cultures are more or less permissive of women's bodies than ours. I become frustrated when people respond to my chagrin over the nipple double standard by saying, "Well at least you're not in a conservative country where you can't even show your ankles." Um, I will not accept that comparison. Don't you dare dangle the plight of women in other countries in front of me as an excuse for why I can't have equal rights in my own country! Should I also be so thankful that I live in a country where we don't allow child brides that I should bow down and be grateful for the gender pay gap? There is a false equivalency here. People everywhere deserve equal rights – just because we might have more rights in some countries than others does not mean we ever should be alright with settling for anything less than equality.

Besides, I could just as easily compare the censorship of women's nipples in America to the high levels of permissiveness of the female body in Europe, where I've frequently seen nude women (and men!) on daytime TV in advertisements and films, with no censorship. These are the same countries where people take their children to nude beaches and this never becomes problematic – because they are teaching their children from a young age that your natural body is *not* a sex object!

Even still, I am so grateful to see the groundswell of sex positive people demanding autonomy over people's bodies sweeping across America, from the well-attended Women's Marches for equality in 2018 and 2019, to the highest number of female lawmakers ever elected to Congress in November

2018. Many US cities, like my home city of Denver, have amended the law to allow (or, "decriminalize" if you will) female toplessness, reducing the shame and stigma of a woman baring her body just like a man. Maybe people fail to realize that this is an autonomy and human rights issue. Women are not protesting to "free the nipple" because they want to walk around topless everywhere and to traumatize and corrupt the minds of impressionable young boys. Rather, we are just trying to get the point across that our bodies are not objects. Sounds reasonable, no?

Circumcision

An interesting example of parents conditioning their children's sexuality surrounds infant male circumcision in America. While the American Association of Pediatrics has repeatedly stated that the medical benefits of male infant circumcision are questionable at best, the practice nonetheless remains rather frequent, especially amongst male parents who were circumcised themselves. This is an example of socially conditioned practice that has a direct effect upon the physical genitals and sexual sensation of boys and men. While the circumcision rate for infants declined from about eight out of ten men in the 1960s to one-third in 2009, other statistics show that the overall circumcision rate of all men in the US is between 76 and 92 per cent (whereas the rate in most Western European countries is around 20 per cent).[9] Young people tend to be much more sceptical of circumcision than older adults. One 2018 poll showed that only around one-third of 18- to 29-year-olds in America would circumcise their male children compared with two-thirds of seniors.[10] Whether the phasing out of the practice has more to do with concerns over the damage of male circumcision or our rejection of conservatism and/or religion remains to be seen. It is also unclear whether men who have been circumcised will expect to do the same to their baby boys.

Media and Body Image

While androgyny has always been popular in fashion, lately gender fluidity has taken the fashion world by storm, with multiple large fashion houses incorporating transgender and gender fluid models into their shows and campaigns, as well as drag queens. In January 2019, Gucci launched *The Future is Fluid* film and campaign, which embraces gender fluidity and the freedom to live as the gender you choose to be. Rihanna's lingerie line, "Savage X Fenty", is set to surpass Victoria's Secret in popularity, mostly because it offers a huge range of sizes to accommodate all women. Indeed, objections to Victoria's Secret's lack of body positive sizing and their narrow view of the "attractive" female body have been rife, with multiple protests staged at their London and New York stores. Popular culture has also been flooded with controversies about body image, with everything from celebrities Photoshopping their Instagram photos, to skincare lines "blackfacing" their models. The most important take-home message here is that maybe for the first time ever, we are waking up to the truth that we are being sold to and we have the opportunity to vote with our dollars. Across social media and beyond, we are demanding a media reality that at least somewhat reflects our actual reality in exchange for our consent to buy the products.

Just as I grew up in the 1990s conditioned to heroin-chic impossibly skinny-looking women (like Kate Moss in her heyday), nowadays the new norm (although no less attainable) is the Kardashian-style "thicc" body with big boobs, big booty and a tiny waist. At least women aren't being asked to shrink themselves down anymore, but this body type is no less sexualized or difficult to attain, with butt implants and lip injections at an all-time high. In fact, the trend of illegal silicone butt injections (usually taking place at "pumping parties" at people's homes) has created dangerous health problems for some women on their quest to attain that giant booty. Jameela Jamil's *I Weigh* initiative has turned heads on social media, positing that what we "weigh" should incorporate the sum of our values as a human being, not just a number on a scale. Her premise is that we never ask about what men weigh, only women, with the goal of shrinking that number on the scale (and shrinking our metaphorical power in the process). These movements reflect the importance of a wide range of body types being accessible in our media, from plus-sized models Hunter McGrady and Ashley Graham starring in the *Sports Illustrated* Swim Suit Editions in 2018 and 2019, to musician and plus-sized activist Lizzo being featured in *Playboy Magazine* (as well as her album going to #1 on the *Billboard* charts), people of all genders are seeking out depictions of beauty that celebrate a wide range of body types and ethnicities.

As an aside, a lot of people ask me what I think about celebrities modifying and selling their bodies as a route to become rich and famous, and honestly, I don't care. Who is anyone to judge them, really? As a sex positive person, I believe that what anyone does with their body is their right only! The most important thing about having a sex positive body image is that you are entitled to love your body right now, and you also are entitled to change the things you don't like or improve yourself however you want.

While we're on this topic … is there really anything wrong with plastic surgery so long as people are present and connected with why they are doing it? Do people take it too far? Sometimes, especially when sketchy procedures are done illegally. But if you really don't like something about your body, being sex positive means you have the right to change it if you want. On the other hand, ask yourself: Will changing this really make me happy? Why it is that you hate this thing about yourself to begin with? Is it really that bad, or is it just social conditioning? Does it really matter in the grand scheme of your life? Being sex positive, where do we draw the line? Most of us do things to make ourselves feel more attractive. Maybe some people want to take more extreme measures. Who cares? Does it really affect us? Can we please not lose sight of the inner beauty of people of all genders, including those who are gender fluid, because body shaming and trolling is ugly. Acceptance of others is not relieving yourself of responsibility; it is an attitude supporting people to create the life and the identity that they choose, yourself included.

After my hysterectomy, I gained closed to 30 pounds in only a few months when my body went into a kind of hormonal shock. For a long time, I felt terrible about myself because of the weight gain and was desperate to lose the weight and get back to where I was before getting sick. At some point I realized that there was no going back to what my body was before the traumatic crisis – all I could do was move forward. Instead of hating my new body, I made a choice to love my new body because it has kept me alive. So rather than starving myself, over-exercising, or finding myself trapped in a negative self-dialogue every time I looked in the mirror, I began to practise gratitude for this body and tell it, *thank you* for being my vessel (or, my flesh suit, haha) that has kept me here in this form. I know this body is far from "perfect" (in the fake news socially conditioned context, at least), but it is the only one I have and I'm going to feel proud of it! It is already enough, even when I decide to work on it to make it stronger or more beautiful.

Last year, I got really into strength training, which gave me back a lot of my confidence because I was so weak when I became ill that I could barely run or lift a five-pound dumbbell. Now, I can run, spin, squat, bench and even lift with heavy weights. Building my muscles back up and increasing the strength in my body has helped me cultivate gratitude for what this body and mind can accomplish. Maybe you've experienced something similar? Even now, six years later, I'm still 20 pounds heavier than I was before my surgery, but I feel 100 per cent stronger and healthier. Seeing a lower number on the scale wouldn't change how I feel about myself. I'm sharing this story because I want you to know that all of us feel unworthy to the extent that we internalize the fake news stories about who we ought to be.

Don't Forget Your Sexual Health!

This includes practising safe sex (by using fluid barriers like condoms, dental dams, spermicidal lube and even latex gloves on some occasions), encouraging the people in our lives to understand and respect consent, seeking out sound medical advice when it comes to hormone therapies and birth control (including asking your doctor: Is this IUD right for me? Should I still be on the pill after ten years? What are the risks of having a vasectomy?), getting regular STI (sexually transmitted infection) screenings, including urine analysis, a blood test and Pap (cervical) smears for women / urethral swabs for men, as well as regular health checks (breast or testicular exams, and so on). Many of these procedures are covered by insurance in the US or covered by health care provision in other Western countries. Even though it may require a little bit of extra effort and time, as sex positive people we are happy to do this because we love our bodies and want them to be as healthy as possible!

Toxic Masculinity (It Hurts Men Too!)

We should not forget that men have traditionally had a bad deal when it comes to gender stereotypes. The hegemonic myth teaches children and adolescents that men are predatory, violent and aggressive – and some of them end up growing up and embodying this narrative. But not everyone does. As alluded to earlier, the extent to which these stereotypes create a self-fulfilling prophecy remains unclear. You've probably heard the term *toxic masculinity* being thrown around as one of the key assailants in the #MeToo movement. Toxic masculinity highlights elements of the hegemonic myth of masculinity, such as misogyny, homophobia, violence and domination. The Good Men Project, an organization dedicated to creating a dialogue about what it means to be a good man in the 21st century, defines toxic masculinity as:

A narrow and repressive description of manhood, designating manhood as defined by violence, sex, status and aggression. It's the cultural ideal of manliness, where strength is everything while emotions are a weakness; where sex and brutality are yardsticks by which men are measured, while supposedly "feminine" traits – which can range from emotional vulnerability to simply not being hypersexual – are the means by which your status as "man" can be taken away.[11]

It is clear that toxic masculinity does not reflect all masculinity and that the gender stereotypes it embodies have become terribly harmful to men as well, including the idea that a man who shows emotion or is sensitive is somehow less than a man; the notion that a real man has to be the "breadwinner"; the belief that real men cannot or should not be feminists; and the misconception that real men should always have an erection and be ready for sex.

Men have always been penalized for failing to adhere to social norms about masculinity to the same extent as women and femininity, if not more. For example, a 2018 study published in the *American Journal of Men's Health* examined the relationship between rigid adherence to norms of hegemonic masculinity and undesirable outcomes like depression, aggression, hostility, self-injury and poor psychological wellbeing. They found that men who felt overly constrained by their gender, and who feared being shamed for not being "masculine" enough, had an increased likelihood of releasing repressed tensions in self-harming ways including increased risk-taking and self-damaging behaviours. Why? Being unable to express their emotions without being shamed, these men sought self-control and self-regulation in the only way they could, by causing harm to themselves as a channel to release their negative emotions.

Most psychologists will tell you that toxic masculinity is as toxic to men as it is to the rest of society. In the age of #MeToo when many people (arguably, fairly) blame toxic masculinity (or at least those who seemingly embody it) for the harassment and assault of women in our society, we must remember that those who are ascribing to such norms may be doing so out of conditioning and may be suffering terribly. On a larger scale, there are *many* men who are actively fighting against toxic masculinity, who do not adhere to these gender roles and who are huge supporters of women. Women are also lending support to those men to help them set an example for others who continue to struggle to overcome the conditioning of a narrow gender identity.

Where Do Our Programmed Sexual Attitudes Come From?

Now that we're familiar with the various norms about gender that we are taught as inherent "truths", as we redefine our attitudes, we must do deep work to trace back the sources of this fake news so that we can begin to consciously replace it with something better. Gender stereotypes come from a variety of sources including our families, the education system, religion, and mass media. Let's examine a little bit about what these institutions might have taught you about yourself so that you can continue to separate the fake old news from the truth about who you are.

Family

Socialization happens from an early age in the context of the family. Children will often unconsciously model everything, from their parents' gender roles to their parents' relationship styles, hang-ups and dysfunctions. Children are often rewarded through conditioning by their parents positively reinforcing certain behaviours while punishing other behaviours. For example, parents frequently allow boys to participate in *rough and tumble play* but often admonish girls from partaking in the same playground behaviours. In psychology, we talk a lot about the power of parents to programme their children's beliefs due to the family's shared genetics and environment. Not only are you likely to behave similarly to your parents (genetics), but you share your home, as well as the cultural institutions in which you participate (environment). Remember the nature versus nurture debate discussed earlier? Your family accounts for both sides of that debate. And even if you were adopted, you will still model your adoptive parents' behaviours.

What are parents teaching their kids about sex? A 2019 survey showed that 1 in 10 adults did not want to discuss gender identity with their children at all, with nearly that many not wanting to discuss sexual orientation either (compare this with only 3 per cent who did not want to discuss sex). There was also more pressure for boys to conform to their gender roles than girls, with three-quarters saying it was ok for their daughter to wear boy's clothes, but less than half believing it was ok for their son to wear a dress.[12] What did your parents teach you about sex and gender? Which of their behaviours are you still modelling as an adult, and which ones no longer serve you?

Education System

The education system is responsible for our formal learning, but it also helps to reinforce many of the ideas about gender and sex that we are taught at a young age. Ideas like the sexual double standard and the objectification of women's clothing choices are especially poignant at school (at least, they were for me). Despite being a straight-A student, I was repeatedly sent to the principal's office because the colour of my tights did not conform to the dress code. Well, technically, the appropriate colour of a girl's tights was not actually specified in the dress code, so I wore every neon colour I could find until they amended the dress code on my behalf. School is the staging space for many of the changes we experience in adolescence and often educators try, but do not do the best job, to support us when we go through puberty. Given the cited research studies that gender norms are internalized as early as age ten, it is good to see more schools putting programmes in place to help combat gender stereotypes, bullying, homophobia, transphobia and sexism. Maybe we should consider dedicating full-term courses to subjects like safe sex, consent and gender identity? (Who really needs to learn calculus, anyway?)

Many parents also expect that the school system will teach their children about safe sex, gender identity and sexual orientation. Yet one of the most interesting issues in American sex education is that, depending upon their districts, some schools have traditionally taught *abstinence only* sex education where there has not been funding available to public schools who teach about intercourse. When I began teaching psychology of sex to college students back in 2004, most of my students knew little about the subject and had a never had a proper sex education course beyond what they learned in one or two days of their health classes. Thankfully this is changing, but America has a long way to go to catch up with European countries, many of which start teaching about gender identity and sexual orientation as early as kindergarten.

Religion

The three major religions in the West (Christianity, Judaism and Islam) take a rather conservative approach to sexuality. Depending upon the religion, this can mean teaching no sex until marriage, that same-sex sexuality is sinful, that sex outside of marriage is forbidden, or that sexuality is something shameful and wrong, and so on. Considering that America is still very much a Christian nation (more than 70 per cent), we can assume that many people, maybe even those reading this book, were raised with a certain amount of religious guilt and shame about their sexuality, especially if they are also LGBTQ+.

There is nothing "wrong" with organized religion, but I do have a personal problem with any dogma, religious or otherwise, that seeks to control and constrain people in ways that make them feel bad or wrong about who they are. Telling anyone that they are going to HELL just for loving who they choose does not sit well with me. We simply have too much evidence of young LGBTQ+ people feeling afraid to come out to their families for fear of judgement, emotional abuse or physical retaliation. Kids and teens who out themselves or are outed by others sometimes end up being beaten, kicked out of the house, or thrown into gay conversion therapy. Yet there is also evidence of individuals raised in religious homes who had families that supported and embraced their alternative sexuality. Based on your religious affiliation, you might have grown up feeling like you were a sinner just for being yourself, which is not acceptable.

Gay Conversion Therapy

Gay conversion therapy (also sometimes known as reparative therapy) is one of the religious elements that has been cruel and downright damaging to our abilities to live sex positive lives. Usually promoted by "Ex-Gay Ministry" religious groups, conversion therapy attempts to eliminate individuals' sexual desires for members of their own sex. Sending young people to "therapy" (in quotes because scientists do not accept this as a form of actual therapy) that tells them that they are wrong about their sexual orientation has been proven to enhance feelings of trauma, fear and self-hatred.[13] Multiple US-based mental health organizations condemn this practice,[14] and yet it continues to be aggressively promoted to the public by political and religious groups. In 2015, the Obama administration supported a ban on gay conversion therapy for minors, with senior advisor Valerie Jarrett saying:

> The overwhelming scientific evidence demonstrates that conversion therapy, especially when it is practiced on young people, is neither medically nor ethically appropriate and can cause substantial harm.[15]

No matter your religion or sexual orientation, being sex positive means rejecting the idea that you are "wrong" when you express your feelings, sexual or otherwise. Everybody must be free to love who they choose, no exceptions. The threat of eternal damnation for loving who you love is the embodiment of hate, not God's love. If you believe in a spirit, or God, or even the flying spaghetti monster, then consider that you were made the way you are for a reason: You are already perfect! You were made out of love, and your natural feelings and desires are something to take pride in, not feel shame over.

Mass Media

Despite what certain corporations might want to you to believe, the mass media's portrayals of love, sex and relationships have never intended to be factual or informative. Television, magazines, films and even social media offer services designed to exploit and entertain, and most notably, to sell us products. Considering that 90 per cent of the mainstream mass media is owned by the same six companies, our access to information is constantly being guided and skewed by the perspectives and information that they want us to see. Even our social media feeds have been completely taken over by advertising disguised as posts that should belong there. It is easy to believe that the media portrayals reflect real life, but often, they are the ultimate social construction designed to make us insecure to sell us products. Just think about the $40 billion per year beauty industry: Could it be they might want you to feel like crap so you buy whatever cream/food plan/pill/accessory might make you love yourself just a little bit more?

Am I being cynical? Maybe. But we have certainly grown up with so many gender stereotypes propagated by children's cartoons about women needing to be rescued (the same hegemonic myth all over again, shocking!) and more broadly, endless amounts of media portrayals showing how a woman's worth lies in her youth and beauty and not in her abilities as a leader. We have been bombarded with warped idealistic visions of toxic masculinity in mainstream action films featuring countless men in starring roles with buff bodies and dominant violent attitudes. Still, it appears that we are beginning to demand more accurate, positive body images, and we are starting to see the first echoes of it reflected in our mass media.

Consider the multiple campaigns for body positivity and embracing all women's body sizes, ages and ethnicities. Beauty giant Unilever has announced its efforts to "change harmful gender norms" and has been at the forefront of body positivity since its Dove adverts launched a few years ago. No discussion here could be complete without mentioning Gillette's 2019 advert asking men to do "*better*" and to hold each other accountable when it comes to bullying, the harassment of women and anti-gay prejudice. This was viewed tens of millions of times when it first came out in early 2019. Gillette, who has traditionally used the copy, "the best a man can get", reframed their brand asking men to "be the best men can be". Some men were offended, feeling that they didn't need a brand or an ad telling them how to be a good man. But given the state of toxic masculinity over the past few years, others disagreed.

We each have the power to reject these stories and write better ones to take their place. A huge part of redefining these attitudes comes from the way we are saying "screw fake news!" by loving ourselves more completely and by starting to reject the idea of gender altogether.

CHAPTER 2

A GENDER FLUID WORLD

Gender Identity and Fluidity

When it comes to redefining love, sex and relationships, there is no issue more relevant or contentious than our generation's rejection of the masculine/feminine gender binary in favour of something more fluid.

Some of us are opening up to gender non-conformity by embracing more fluid presentations of our gender when it comes to hairstyle and clothing. Others are feeling more comfortable than ever with *cross-gender roles*, like women working in the sciences or men staying at home with their children. Still others are taking the rejection of gender norms even further by refusing to participate in the binary at all and self-identifying as something "other" than masculine or feminine. More than ever before, we are turning away from the gender binary and defining ourselves as gender neutral, gender queer, gender fluid, or transgender (we'll talk about the psychology of these terms a little bit later on in the chapter).

Unless you've been living in an apocalyptic bunker since 2000, you've no doubt been exposed to myriad opinions, headlines and pieces of legislation addressing individuals who choose to live as something other than the sex they were assigned to at birth. Rejecting the idea of gender as a binary – seeing only two genders, male and female – has taken up a massive space in the political sphere, from the transgender bathroom debate, to attempts to ban transgendered people from serving in the US military, to some states now offering alternative genders on drivers' licences, to Facebook now permitting over 50 potential choices for your gender identity besides "*male*" and "*female*".

Millennials and Generation-Z (broadly defined as those born after the year 2000) are much more permissive of gender fluidity than past generations and much more likely to be gender fluid themselves. A 2017 poll conducted by *GLAAD* found that about 1 in 10 millennials in the US identify as transgender or gender fluid, much higher than previous generations.[16] In the 2015 *Fusion Massive Millennial Poll*, over half of millennials believed that gender identity is a spectrum and that "some people fall outside of the conventional categories".[17] In 2019, the Pew Research Center found that roughly equal numbers of millennials and Gen-Z individuals believed that society should be more accepting of people who do not identify as male or female.[18]

In most polls, millennials and Gen-Z generally look nearly identical on key social and political measures. One of the exceptions? People born as Gen-Z are slightly more likely than millennials to know someone who uses a gender-neutral pronoun (and the percentage decreases as you look at older generations).[19] More than one-third of Gen-Z respondents and younger millennials said that gender did not define them as a person as much as it used to, and Gen-Z individuals were also less likely than millennials to only buy clothes designed for their own gender.[20]

The conclusion? Gen-Z individuals might actually be even more "Queer AF" than millennials. While we have even less data on Gen-Z than millennials, as of late, these polls indicate a clear trend of embracing attitudes that reject the gender binary in favour of something more fluid. Traditional attitudes about gender identity no longer define our expressions or destinies as they once did. A recent *Forbes* article even explained how "gender stereotypes are not only outdated but insulting" to many of us, and that the smart brands are listening, marketing a lifestyle based upon personality and expression, rather than a gender, as they once did.[21] Just look at how massive global consumer clothing brands like Zara and H&M have launched successful gender-neutral clothing lines over the past few years, something that would have been almost unheard of just a mere decade ago.

Is gender fluidity a form of identity expression or a sort of resistance against the limiting norms of the patriarchy and the status quo? Depending upon the individual, it could be a bit of both.

A Note about Identity Labels

Transgender visibility has absolutely sky-rocketed in the past ten years across politics, social media and amongst our friends and loved ones, but a lack of clarity about the many types of transgendered identities persists, often leading to confusion, anger and discrimination. It is important for us to get on the same page so that together, we can establish mutual understanding and respect for one another. Indeed, sex positive attitudes include accepting people's right to choose how to represent their gender identities, recognizing the choice to be gender fluid and the many obstacles and challenges that people face along the way.

Humans naturally turn to labels and categories to store, organize and recall information. One size does not fit all, and many of the labels that we use to categorize sexuality can become exclusionary, inaccurate and problematic. Nonetheless, it is only through some semblance of shared language that we can collectively become more conscious about everyone's sexual choices.

I encourage you to reject any label or category that does not apply to your identity, and, most importantly, to remain flexible since these categories are constantly evolving and being revised as people explore their identities more deeply. Many of these new labels for gender identity barely existed in psychology or slang when I began teaching human sexuality over a decade ago. It is up to you to build the identity that best serves your development as a sex positive person.

Gender Psychology

For too long, gender has been associated with whatever someone is packing in between their legs. Yet any psychologist will tell you that gender is a *social construct* that has everything to do with how masculine or feminine we feel inside and how we intend for the world to perceive us. It has nothing to do with our sex chromosomes, physical anatomy or biological sex. It also has *nothing* to do with your sexual orientation toward who you might fall in love with, date or have sex with.

If we wind the clock back 50 years, gender would have been considered in mainstream narrative as the same as *biological sex*, referring to the genitals you were born with. We each get an X chromosome from our mothers and an X or Y chromosome from our fathers, although sometimes people are born intersexed, meaning they have something other than XX or XY. Let's say a child named Andrew is born is with a penis and XY chromosomes. We would call XY his *chromosomal sex* – XX for women, XY for men, as well as variation in people who are born XO, XXY, and so on. When Andrew is born, the doctor slaps him on the behind and says, "It's boy!!!" This would then be his *assigned sex.*[22]

Gender identity is defined in psychology as a person's deeply felt, inherent sense of being a boy, a man, or male; a girl, a woman, or female; or an alternative gender (such as genderqueer, gender non-conforming, gender neutral) that may or may not correspond to a person's sex assigned at birth or to a person's primary or secondary sex characteristics.[23] Returning to our simple example, Andrew might grow up with a masculine gender identity, meaning that his inherent sense of identity is *normative* because his biological sex and his gender identity match up. (This doesn't mean that he would inherently embody toxic masculinity, though!) We would call Andrew a *cisgender* person, which describes a person whose gender identity and gender expression align with their assigned sex at birth. We could also call him a *chromosomal male* because his gender and chromosomes match. Some people prefer this term to cisgender.

So far, Andrew's example sounds fairly typical, harkening back to the narrative of cisgender identities that are commonly portrayed to us through mainstream media. However, Andrew may have embarked upon a different journey to express his gender identity. Maybe as a child, he was naturally drawn to playing with dolls instead of toy cars and took a liking to wearing dresses. He may have always felt inside that he was meant to be born as a woman, identifying more deeply with a feminine gender identity. In this case, a psychologist may have diagnosed him as having *gender dysphoria*, which is defined as *a conflict between a person's biological sex or assigned gender and the gender with which he/she/they identify*. People with gender dysphoria can feel distress at their bodies (particularly during the changes that happen in puberty) as well as with the roles that are assigned to their gender. This distress can lead them to pursue treatment ranging from psychotherapy, to altering how they present their gender, to the use of hormones to modify perceived undesirable masculine or feminine characteristics, to full-on sex reassignment surgery. However, not everyone with gender dysphoria seeks out these treatments, and some abstain from all therapies entirely.

Let's say that Andrew decides he wants to become Annie, adopting a female gender pronoun and feminine gender identity. This would make Andrew *transgender* or *gender fluid* because his gender identity differs from his assigned sex, biological sex and/or chromosomal sex. This is regardless of whether he has sex reassignment surgery or pursues other treatments to bring his physical body into alignment with his gender identity.

According to census data analysed by researchers at UCLA, about 0.5 per cent or 1.4 million adults in the US identify as transgender (individuals aged 18 to 24 are the adults most likely to self-identify as such).[24] Because of the still present stigma over being transgender, some respondents may have declined to report their gender identity, meaning that these numbers could actually be much higher. For example, researchers at the Boston

University School of Medicine have argued that disorders of gender identity affect as many as 1 in 100 people, with another poll showing that about 1 in 6 of millennials feel that their gender identity differs from the sex they were assigned at birth.[25]

If Annie wanted to have full-on sex reassignment surgery to replace her penis with a vagina, then in the past she would have been labelled *transsexual*, although this terminology is being phased out. In the US, as many as 1 out of 30,000 adult males seek sexual reassignment surgery annually, and at least 1 out of 100,000 adult females.

This is where our story gets even more complicated. One of the most challenging parts of unpacking gender identity is that the term "transgender" serves as an umbrella term including not only people who are seeking to transition from one gender or sex to the other, but also people who do not *exclusively* identify as one gender or the other. The term *transgender** (with an asterisk) is sometimes used to describe all people who reject a cisgender or chromosomal model of gender.

What if Andrew did not necessarily identify as a woman or seek to undergo a *gender transition*? What if he felt more like he was *gender non-binary, genderqueer* or maybe he rejected gender altogether?

Gender fluidity, also known as *gender non-binary* or *genderqueer*, is a catchall category that refers to people with gender identities that are not exclusively masculine or feminine, falling outside of the binary (or cisnormative) gender categories of "male" and "female".

This is where many of our labels and preconceived notions start to break down. Being gender non-binary could reflect a variety of distinct identities: A person could feel an overlap of masculine and feminine identities but no desire to choose to identify with one or the other; they might be gender fluid (meaning they have a fluctuating gender identity); they could also reject gender or have no gender (being agender, non-gender or genderless); or they could have multiple genders (making them bigender, trigender or pangendered).

When actress and activist Ruby Rose explained her specific feelings on her own gender fluidity in 2014, she was one of the first public figures to address the concept:

Gender fluidity is not really feeling like you're at one end of the spectrum or the other. For the most part, I definitely don't identify as any gender. I'm not a guy; I don't really feel like a woman, but obviously I was born one. So, I'm somewhere in the middle, which – in my perfect imagination – is like having the best of both sexes. I have a lot of characteristics that would normally be present in a guy and then less that would be present in a woman. But then sometimes I'll put on a skirt – like today. The takeaway is that only you know who you were born to be, and you need to be free to be that person.[26]

Anyone who does not conform to one of the two gender categories could find themselves identifying as genderqueer, but they might feel totally different from someone who identifies as transgender. A genderqueer person may be content fluctuating across both genders or living as a different gender entirely, whereas a transgender person may specifically seek to transition from one gender to the other. Adding to our confusion is the fact that being genderqueer, gender fluid or gender non-binary also does not necessarily meet the psychological diagnostic criteria for having gender dysphoria – because there is difference between feeling like you were born in the wrong physical body (gender dysphoria), and feeling like your society's instructive labels don't apply to your unique expression of your identity (genderqueer or gender fluid). More and more, people are embracing the idea of gender as social construct and refusing to be categorized altogether.

Returning to our simplified example, instead of transitioning to become Annie, Andrew might identify as gender non-binary, and in rejection of the binary decide to change gender pronouns from he/his/mr to ze/zey/zir. The importance of using the correct pronouns has become so relevant that many colleges are making strides to ensure that students have options to articulate the pronoun that best suits their gender identity. According to Jessica Bennet, the gender editor of the *New York Times*, introducing your gender pronoun on a college campus happens in the same way that you would tell people your major. So instead of saying, "Hi, this is my name, and this is my major," I might say, "Hi, I'm Kelly, my pronouns are she/her/hers and my major is psychology." Some of the potential gender pronouns being used across college campuses include "E" at Harvard, "ey" at American University, "hir" (a combination of his and her), "xe" or "ve" or "ne" or "per" (for person), or "thon" (a blend of "that" and "one") or "Mx", an alternative to Ms and Mr.[27]

Representations of gender fluidity have made a huge splash not only on Instagram but all the way across the mainstream media. We're seeing celebrities showing up on red carpets in outfits that include elements that are traditionally associated with men's clothing (ties, suit coats), blended with ones traditionally associated with women (skirts, high heels). Television has grown rife with representations of transgender characters, actors and storylines that embody gender fluidity. Being gender fluid is no longer a hidden fringe experience: It is becoming part of the mainstream fabric of our daily lives.

With new characterizations of gender identity constantly emerging, it can be really hard to keep track of the correct language, even for people working in the field of sexology like myself. Many people who are cisgender have reported feeling alienated and confused about these new identities, just as people who ascribe to them often feel rejected and judged by the mainstream. Perhaps the take-home lesson here is for everyone to chill and allow people to self-identify their genders in the way that makes the most sense for their sex positive lives. Listen to people when they tell you who they are. If someone else doesn't like your gender pronoun, that's fine because it really has nothing to do with them anyway. And if someone refuses to acknowledge the pronoun of your choice, there's not much you can do except to keep your head up, stick to your guns and maybe burn down their house (I'm kidding).

How the Past Can Inform the Future

With the acceptance of gender fluidity at an all-time high in our brave new world, it can be easy to forget that the possibility of living outside of the gender binary has always been an acceptable option throughout many cultures in human history. This isn't a new idea, although the individuals who call us "snowflakes" make it sound as though we are reinventing the wheel. We're not. Some cultures have as many as third, fourth and fifth genders. People living outside of the binary gender have not always been marginalized the way that they have been in Western society over the last few centuries. Since we must look to the past to understand the future, so please consider the following anecdotes from history.

"*Two-Spirits*", or, third gender Native Americans have existed for centuries, according to Lakota two-spirit artist and activist Centazi Nicholas Metcalf, who gave a Ted Talk on the topic in 2015.[28] He argues that of 556 indigenous tribal communities, nearly all of them have documentation of two-spirit or transgendered persons (in this case, "two-spirit" refers to an individual who embodies both male and female characteristics). Rather than being shunned, two-spirits have been traditionally valued by their tribal communities, considered story-tellers who can teach sacred ceremonies. Two-spirits are also considered "sacred bridge builders" between the masculine and feminine, and tribal myths even characterize them as saving our world – an interesting concept considering that this epoch of the many challenges facing humanity's survival is the time when the transgender equality movement has become the most visible to the mainstream.

Notions similar to the two-spirits have been documented in indigenous cultures across Hawaii, Madagascar, South America and Asia. One contemporary example of ancient transgender acceptance that still exists today are the *"Hijra"* in India. Not a country known for its progressive stance on sexuality, India has nonetheless recognized the sacredness of the third gender hijra population, who have enjoyed more freedom and recognition than the country's lesbian, gay and bisexual population in recent times no doubt owed to their vast historical significance. For over 4,000 years since the ancient literature of *Kama Sutra*, the hijra (broadly defined as India's transgender male to female population) have been recognized as sacred religious beings in some of the most important texts in Hinduism, including the *Mahabharata* and *Ramayana*. While British colonial rule tried to eradicate and criminalize them, the hijra nonetheless were celebrated during Indian independence.

I could go on, but you can research for yourself to understand the rich and varied global history of transgender people. All the way from the Greek myths of hermaphrodite (who was deemed to possess ultimate insight by way of having both male and female wisdom) to the current-day recognition of two-spirits and hijra as sacred beings, being transgender is definitely much more than a new concept designed for "attention".

What Is NORMAL, Anyway?

If you're like me, you're probably wondering, why do so many cisgender feel violated and angry about transgender people? Particularly those who have little to no access to actual transgender individuals? Are we just naturally uncomfortable with people and situations we don't understand?

It would appear that the collapse of the male/female gender binary is a red flag for everyone holding onto the outdated status quo about sex and relationships. Many people, particularly older adults approaching the third decade of the 21st century, are recoiling in horror at the mere concept that someone could reject their biological or assigned sex in favour of something that felt more comfortable or (gasp) *normal* to them. Yes, there might still be many people out there who believe that transgender people are "freaks, weirdos or sickos". But as sex positive people, we must regard the visibility of the transgender* and allies' movement as a sign that we are breaking down these crusty old views about sex and relationships and redefining them with something more diverse and, certainly, more inclusive.

When it comes to human sexuality, *there is no such thing as normal.* Yes, there are statistical norms (like averages), but there is no moral "right or wrong" normal, so long as you are not causing harm without consent to yourself or to someone else. As a seasoned sex educator, I learned this lesson the hard way, when I'd have lines of students out the door after every class asking if there was something "wrong" with them or if they were in fact "normal". During my first year of teaching I had to take a break from my course syllabus so that I could explain the facts about this so-called normality we are all chasing. I used to tell my classes that there is no difference in "normality" (barring statistical average of course) between a person who masturbates once in 30 years, and a person who masturbates 30 times per day. They are both "normal" in the eyes of sexual science, just like a person who wants to change their gender or live as gender fluid. Even as early as the 1950s, Kinsey taught us that the range of human sexual behaviour is far greater than we could ever imagine.[29] We cannot afford to pathologize the variation in our species just because it no longer fits into what our institutions have conditioned us to believe in the past was morally "right" or "wrong".

Just as Carl Jung said that "*to be normal is the ultimate aim of the unsuccessful,*" being sex positive means that we accept how we all exist as expressions of the wide variation of human behaviour, including but not limited to gender, sexual orientation, the sexual body, kinks, relationship styles and so on. There is a liberation in allowing other people the same freedoms that you want for yourself. So how can we understand the lingering fears about transgender people perpetuated by society at large? Why the urge to ban transgender people from the military, or from public bathrooms, or from expressing their gender transitions or a third gender on their state identifications?

The Distinctiveness Threat Hypothesis

One of the key underlying factors here is that being transgender greatly disrupts the perception of a simple right and wrong approach to sexuality. Since even before the birth of Christianity 2,000 years ago, the way to dominate a society has been through controlling people's relationships, their ability to procreate as well as their perception of their sexual bodies. As more and more people begin to reject the notion of sexuality as a shameful, hidden exclusionary experience, perhaps those who still ascribe to the traditional model of gender and sex feel that their way of life is being threatened.

Maybe this level of dissonance over the violation of the categories that we use to define our world is enough to make people wary or hateful toward transgendered individuals. According to *social identity theory* in psychology, the groups to which we belong help to define our own identities. When the categories of these groups are blurred, we can experience what psychologists call a *"distinctiveness threat"* where we suddenly become unsure of who we are because the boundaries of the group definitions have become too malleable. We no longer feel distinct or unique because the metric we used to define ourselves has crumbled away. Since many people do define themselves according to gender and the norms and roles associated with gender (the clothes we wear, the activities in which we participate, as we discussed in the previous chapter), it would make sense that people who disrupt these deeply held categories would garner a certain amount of rage and dislike.

While psychological research on this topic is incredibly new, a 2018 study published in the journal *Sex Roles* sought to determine whether the distinctiveness threat hypothesis was real and which type of gender non-conformity was more violating to people who value the gender binary: a cisgender person or a transgender person. The researchers ran three studies asking a total of nearly 1,000 participants to read stories about hypothetical individuals who were either cisgender or transgender, and who were either gender conforming or non-conforming. Overall, they found that participants liked the gender conforming and cisgender individuals more, and they perceived the transgender and gender non-conforming individuals as more threatening to the distinction between men and women.

The most interesting finding in this study was that of all four categories (gender-conforming cisgender, gender conforming transgender, gender non-conforming cisgender and gender non-conforming transgender) the group that was perceived as most threatening was the *gender conforming transgender group*: Transgender individuals who conformed to the traditional binary gender role associated with their gender expressions (such as a transgender man who became a woman and then conformed to women's gender roles). Although it may perhaps seem counterintuitive, this finding makes perfect sense in light of the distinctiveness threat hypothesis. If you still ascribe to the gender binary and feel that being a woman or a man is central to your identity, then being presented with someone who was born as one gender but passes as the other is especially threatening. As the researchers observed, "it is likely that conforming transgender individuals (because they can 'pass' as their authentic gender) are especially threatening because they provide some evidence that there are more than two binary genders, or that [one's] binary gender can be changed."[30] Transgender people successfully "passing" as the opposite gender basically proves that gender is a fluid social construct, taking a giant metaphorical dump on those adhere to a strict gender binary.

It is important to remember that it is never a transgender person's fault that people respond vitriolically to their identity choices. As a *Psychology Today* write-up on this study explains, "Transprejudice stems from an internal process in which the person holding the prejudice experiences a threat to an aspect of their own identity, and thus lashes out against trans individuals as a means of trying to reaffirm the boundaries surrounding important aspects of how they define their identity – in this case, their gender."[31]

Mythbusters: Transgender Edition

If a man comes across a transgender woman who can be just as much of a "man" as he is, what does this mean for his identity as a man? This is the essence of distinctiveness threat. The solution? Working together to reduce *gender essentialist beliefs* (the belief that the gender binary is real). Our generation has already begun embracing tolerance and leading by example. We can also exhibit more compassion for those who are being discriminated against, as well as for those who are causing the discrimination out of their own fears and deeply held insecurities. Furthermore, we can lend a story and a voice to all people who are seeking to live more fluid lives by refuting the following myths whenever we hear them.

Myth 1: Transgender People Are Out to Trick and Mislead
Trans activist German Lopez identifies the "number one" transgender myth: That transgender people are somehow confused and tricking or misleading others.[32] This myth, which is "baffling to a lot of transgender people" (according to Mara Keisling, a trans woman and executive director of the National Centre of Transgender Equality), appears to be responsible for phobic attitudes and distrust of transgender individuals. The statistics are not particularly heartening: According to a 2016 poll, about 1 in 5 adults in the US said they would not want to befriend or date a transgendered person, although millennials were much more favourable about befriending and dating transgendered people than older adults.[33]

Interestingly, burgeoning research suggests that not only are transgender people *not* confused, but perhaps, there may be a biological marker for their gender identity. Researchers from Boston University Medical Center recently conducted a review on the available literature on transgender identities, suggesting that there may actually be a biological basis in the brain for gender identity.[34] A consortium of five research institutions in Europe and the US (including Vanderbilt, George Washington University and Boston University) are currently looking to the human genome to explain why people assigned one gender so persistently identify with another, often from very early childhood. We are currently awaiting the results of this study, but two decades of brain research shows that, much like sexual orientation, gender identity may have underpinnings in the brain. The researchers are not seeking to produce a genetic test for being transgender, but rather hope for better care and treatment of transgender people, who often experience health disparities when compared with the general population.

Myth 2: Transgender People Are Doing it "For Attention"
Relating to the first myth, one of the myths that I absolutely hate is that transgender people are doing this "for attention" (which people used to say about being gay in the 1990s and who knows, maybe they still do). I find it quite ridiculous that anyone would choose to endure this level of judgement and transition solely for attention. It is possible that maybe some do, but personally and professionally I believe that the overwhelming majority of transgender people are not doing this for attention. Either their pain at their dysmorphia is so great and extreme that they would rather violate society's rules on gender, or they feel they simply cannot abide by the binary any longer. This is a sign of bravery, not cowardice or doing it "for attention". Find me one person who really wants that kind of life-shattering attention from their friends, family and educators. I dare you.

Myth 3: Being Transgender Is the Same as Being Lesbian, Gay or Bisexual
While the T in LGBTQ stands for transgender, being transgender has nothing to do with sexual orientation

the way that being lesbian, gay or bisexual does! One of the biggest confounds that I have seen repeatedly as a sex educator is the incorrect assumption that a person's gender identity dictates their sexual orientation. Put another way, there is a stereotypical, heteronormative binary assumption that a person who manifests female gender traits would be attracted to males, while a person with masculine gender traits should be attracted to females. We know now very clearly in psychology that how masculine, feminine, gender fluid or agender you might be, this has nothing (no correlation whatsoever!) to do with who your sexual or romantic attractions are!

However, we can thank the transgender equality and gender non-binary movements for offering us a new paradigm for looking at sexual orientation. In psychology, sexual orientation is best measured upon a continuum (known as the Kinsey Scale) ranging from fully heterosexual on one side, to fully homosexual on the other side. Most people place somewhere on this spectrum (at least, this was the case ten years ago). If you were bisexual, you placed somewhere in the middle, and if you were more exclusively homosexual or heterosexual, you placed at either end of the spectrum.

The rise of a new type of category of sexual orientation is pushing us to understand sexual orientation in a more inclusive, gender-blind way. Rather than bisexual being the only option (attracted to both men and women) we now have the option of being attracted to multiple gender identities.

Pansexual (or *omnisexual*) refers to the sexual, romantic or emotional attraction to people regardless of their sex or gender identity. Some see this as an alternative and more inclusive perspective than bisexuality, because it includes attraction to not only cisgender men and cisgender women, but also attraction to people who are transgender, gender non-binary, third gender, agender and so on. From celebrities like Miley Cyrus identifying as pansexual, to a variety of sitcoms, shows and films featuring pansexual characters, this new take on sexual orientation is certainly building momentum in popular culture. I have always been bisexual, but now I am questioning whether I am actually pansexual? Yet I have never questioned that my gender identity is female. Do you see the difference? How you feel inside about your identity, and who you are attracted to, are two completely different concepts.

Myth 4: Allowing a Transgender Person to Use the Bathroom of Their Gender Identity Is Dangerous

Naturally, transgender people want to use the bathroom of their gender identity and not the sex that they are assigned at birth. Conservative critics have long argued that this somehow exposes other people to sexual voyeurism and assault, although there is absolutely no evidence of any such claims. In the US, there are over 18 states and hundreds of schools and colleges that allow transgender people to use the bathroom of their gender identities, and no such crimes have *ever* been reported. Still, the debate continues in certain states, prompted by fearmongering that "sexual predators" will somehow manipulate this law to sneak into women's bathrooms and attack women. This whole notion is incredibly insulting to transgender people by lumping them in with sexual predators and assuming that allowing them to use the bathroom of their gender identity somehow legalizes assault, stalking and voyeurism. It doesn't.

The US Transgender Center for Equality explains that private or separate bathrooms are not the answer here, either. Much like the debate over African Americans using the same bathrooms as whites during the Civil Rights Movement, the idea that transgender people should use a separate bathroom continues to breed marginalization and discrimination. Furthermore, in the case of gender fluid or gender non-binary people, choosing the right bathroom can be a challenge – they should be able to use the bathroom that they feel safest in. The majority of millennials in America support transgender people using the bathroom of their gender identity at a rate of 2:1 for people aged 18 to 29, whereas for people over 60 this statistic was reversed, 2:1 in favour of them not using the bathroom of their gender identity.[35]

Myth 5: Transgender People Are the Same as Drag Queens
Some transgender people might be drag queens, and some drag queens might be transgender, but they are definitely not one and the same. Drag represents a form of subversive art where people transform themselves into the opposite gender for the sake of performance, entertainment and social commentary. Drag performance has always manifested itself as a strong representation of queerness and queer culture, as well as a great example of gender-bending, but in the past few years it has certainly evolved into a worldwide mainstream phenomenon. Thanks to programming like *RuPaul's Drag Race*, people across the world have fallen in love with variety drag queen characters known for their style, comedy skills, beauty, lip-sync acumen and makeup abilities. I'm not ashamed to admit that I learned how to properly apply my makeup from watching drag queens (hello, contour and baking!). And in the true spirit of breaking down the gender binary, many male drag queens make some of the most beautiful females I have ever seen. There is something liberating about witnessing the transformation. Interesting how the massive cisgender female fandom of *Drag Race* isn't triggered by distinctiveness threat when we see men portraying women. Maybe it is because it is only performance, or maybe it is because we never really ascribed too strongly to the gender binary to begin with?

The rising popularity of drag queens and drag performance highlights a shift away from clinging to the gender binary and emphasizes our desire and joy in seeing it bent and twisted out of shape. There is something incredibly satisfying and sex positive about seeing something so subversive garnering such mainstream popularity, with drag queens appearing in Oscar-nominated films, haute couture fashion campaigns, the US *Billboard* Hot 100, and their own highly rated television shows. Drag has also helped highlight the intersectionality of artistic performance versus transgender identities. Despite some overlap here, drag serves as a form of subversive art and entertainment whereas being transgender serves as a true identity. Sometimes, transgender people start out doing drag first and then decide they identify with this way of living full time.

Trans Allies

Even with all of the sex positive progress happening, transgender discrimination remains a very real phenomenon and it is something that we will continue to work against as we redefine the meaning of gender. In your quest to bring more sex positivity into your life, please consider also becoming a transgender ally if you are not one already. Allies put the "A" in LGBTQIA+ and offer support to those who are transgender in their lives and communities. Here are a few tips I value for how to become the best sex positive, transpositive ally you can be, and you can find more on GLADD's transgender allies page.[36]

1 *Listen to people when they explain their trans identities*
   Most importantly, the way that trans people self-identify is the way they want to be recognized by others, much like the rest of us. We want the world to see us the way we want to be seen. A transgender person might tell you if they want to be seen as transsexual, genderqueer, non-binary and so on. Please listen. It surprisingly easy to simply ask, "What pronoun do you prefer?" and then listen. Most people who identify as transgender or gender fluid will appreciate the opportunity to be heard. Others may still be unsure, so please be patient with them.

2 *Respect the pronouns a trans person uses to identify themselves*
Following the first point, if someone tells you their
pronoun, then please use it! As we discussed earlier, there are
so many possible gender pronouns out there. Sometimes in
the professional environment, due to fears of discrimination
a transgender person may not get to use the pronoun they
would like, so listen for this dichotomy as well. Other times
a person does not want to use pronouns at all and just wants
to be called by their name. Please, for the love of all things
holy, do not refer to a transgender person as "it" unless that
person has specifically requested that pronoun. These are
basic matters of human rights and identity which we must
respect unless otherwise noted. A person is *never* an it.

3 *Don't ask about a transgender person's genitals, surgeries or sex life*
This is about as private as it gets, and some people you meet
could be in the middle of these transitions and not feel
ready to discuss it with others. Others might want to talk
about it, and others might not. Just like you wouldn't ask a
stranger what they are packing between their legs, the same
applies. Don't ask if they are "pre-op" or "post-op". If they
want to tell you, they will. Everyone transitions differently,
and sometimes these questions can make it seem like there is
a right or wrong way to do it. There isn't.

4 *Don't make assumptions about a transgender person's sexual
orientation*
As mentioned earlier, gender and sexual orientation are not the
same thing. A transgender person can identify as straight, gay,
lesbian, bisexual, pansexual or anything else that a cisgender
person could identify as. Please do not make assumptions and
ask if you are unsure. Also please consider that coming out
as a transgender person is very different and much more life
altering than coming out as gay, lesbian or bisexual.

5 *Be careful about "outing", confidentiality and disclosure*
Just because a person shares their transgender status with
you does not mean they are necessarily ready to share that
status with the world, including their family, colleagues and
employers. If a person shares this status with you, please be
sensitive before sharing with others. Although it is waning,
discrimination against transgender people is still a real
threat in our society. Please think mindfully of this and do
not share someone's transgender status with another person
unless you have permission to speak about it.

6 *Know your limits as an ally*
If you are not transgender, no matter how sensitive or how
connected you are, there is still probably a lot you don't
know. I am not gender fluid, and there are things I could
never possibly know, but I am always open to learn. It is
better to ask questions than to make assumptions, and to be
kind and compassionate whenever possible.

I hope this chapter has helped clarify and redefine much
of the gender fluid world which we are moving into. You can
find more resources in the recommended reading section if you
have questions or if you or someone you know is looking for
support. The previous chapter emphasized the fake news of the
past, and this chapter showed how we are saying *"fuck fake news"*
by embracing gender fluidity. But no discussion of our changing
social landscapes could be complete without a look into the
sexual innovations of the future (which have already begun!):
Hold onto your hats, folks, because we're about to explore how
the *technosexual revolution* is redefining the very nature of love
and sex.

CHAPTER 3
THE TECHNOSEXUAL REVOLUTION

Now that we've uncovered our socially conditioned fake news, let's consider the impact upon redefining love and sex of the most pervasive, all-encompassing element of our modern social lives: Technology. The evolution of sexual technology has already begun to redefine everything we think we know about love, sex and relationships. Innovations in technology offer a unique, exciting, sometimes juicy and often overwhelming time to explore love and sex in this world. From the development of AI sex robots, to sex-doll vacation brothel tourism, to sex workers being paid in bitcoins, to dating sites that tell you exactly how many miles you are from your next "B.J." (blow job), to virtual reality devices that could make you get off so hard (using your brain!) that you may never need to touch yourself or another human again, the technosexual revolution continues to reshape our erotic boundaries in every conceivable direction.

As technology evolves at an exponentially rapid rate, will developments in pornography, virtual partners and sex dolls mean we could soon inhabit a world where two flesh-and-blood humans might no longer be necessary for love, sex and relationships to take place? How can a sex positive person make sense of these rapid changes, and what does the technosexual revolution mean for our current and future understandings of love and sex?

The Technosexual Takeover

Given that the sex-tech industry is worth over $30 billion per year globally,[37] we can rest assured that scientists will continue using their considerable brainpower to tune us in and turn us on. *Sex-tech* itself is generally defined as "technology, and technology-driven ventures, designed to enhance, innovate and disrupt in every area of human sexuality and human sexual experience."[38] This broad definition includes everything from Internet porn, to sex toys, to online dating, webcams, sex dolls and whatever other freaky tech the future may yield. According to this definition, the first type of "sex-tech" was the first erotic films made in the late 19th century in France. It is absolutely astounding (although perhaps not surprising) to see how quickly this industry has evolved to shape so many aspects of modern human sexuality.

It is nearly impossible to predict exactly how the ongoing sex-tech explosion could revolutionize all aspects of human sexuality. The most notable trend with sex-tech is that as soon as technological developments are made, we horny humans can't help but commandeer them for our sexual pleasure. For example, the mass market consumption of sexually explicit films grew rapidly with the invention of 8mm and Super-8 film and cinematography – coinciding with the mass market appeal of erotic magazines in the mid 20th century. By the 1970s, full-length explicit pornographic films were receiving theatrical releases in the US, starting with *Mona the Virgin Nymph* (1970), followed by *Boys in the Sand* (1972), which was the first ever gay pornographic film with a theatrical release, as well as the first to give credits to its cast, the first to be reviewed by the *New York Times* and the first erotic film to parody an existing film. When *Deep Throat* was released in 1972, so many people gagged that it truly solidified pornography as a mainstream social phenomenon, allegedly grossing $1 million during the first month of its release in cinema (the HBO series *The Deuce* does a great job portraying this moment in history).

After 5,000 plus years of sexual depictions and drawings, suddenly within the past 100 years, still photography and actual moving sex pictures have come to dominate our use of erotic materials; but that's not the whole story. Within a few short years from the theatrical release of pornography films, a mere blip on the radar of human evolution, we have seen the rise (and fall) of home video pornography on VHS in the 1980s, as well as the introduction of erotic CD-ROMs in the 1990s that offered enhanced interactive experiences, followed by their subsequent decline as, kaboom! the Internet was born.

The Juggernaut of Internet Porn

The accessibility of the Internet, paired with the digital media revolution of the 21st century, has created a totally unique time in human history integrating high-quality instant streaming video, a seemingly endless variety of erotic images, the ability for anyone to create and upload pornography and instant free access at our fingertips.[39] Gone are the days of sneaking under your parents' bed to look at your dad's *Playboy* stash, "accidentally" buying a dirty movie in a hotel or waiting on dial-up for 13 minutes as you slowly watch a pair of titties load frame-by-frame. Are humans watching more porn than ever now that we have complete, unabated instant access anytime, anywhere? You better believe it. Do we even need the presence of another human being to get off anymore? Not really.

According to some researchers, over one-quarter of all Internet searches and 30 per cent of all data transferred on the Internet is pornographic in nature! Others argue that at least 1 in 10 of all adults on the Internet at any given time are searching for porn.[40] A survey of nearly 1,000 Americans showed that more than 75 per cent of American men and women aged 18 to 30 report watching porn at least once a month.[41] Still, it is difficult to gauge exactly how many people are watching porn at any given time, or how much of the Internet is really composed of pornographic or erotic material because most of the adult industry is privately owned, making it difficult to objectively surmise from a statistical point of view.

Thankfully, individual pornographic websites like PornHub do a fantastic job of tracking user data and sharing it with the public. In its most recent *Year in Review* statistics, PornHub reports using a bandwidth of 4,403 Petabytes or 4,403,000 GB, which is more bandwidth than the entire Internet streamed in 2002![42]

According to PornHub, nearly 9 in 10 college-age men and 1 in 3 college-age women in the US watched porn on their website every single day. Globally, over half of all porn viewers are millennials, which is hardly surprising considering our inherent love for all things technological.

The Psychology of Porn Search Fantasies

The overall trends in porn viewership reflect certain taboos and fantasies that are very different for men and women. Men's top ten searches include "MILF" (Mom I'd Like to Fuck) and "step-mom" while "lesbian" is the most popular with women. This search disparity offers an interesting window into the psychology of pornography use as way to explore fantasies and taboos.

All sorts of naughty, illicit behaviours (cheating, step-family sex, outdoor sex, sex in your parents' bed, etc) can be major turn-ons, but we cannot assume that the men watching MILF or step-mom porn actually want to have sex with their moms! When it comes to MILF porn, when a man feels he has no outlet to express his attractions to older women without being shamed, he may use porn to explore and safely indulge in this fantasy.

Most likely the popularity of MILF porn has less to do with the women actually being "moms" and more to do with how the older women depicted seem confident, knowledgeable about sex and have huge sexual appetites. Rather than being innocent and needing to be led or taught, the women in MILF porn know exactly how to get themselves off, as well as their younger male partners. The level of power and dominance possessed by the women in MILF/step-mom porn is substantially more than women in regular 18+ porn, at least according to a study published in the *Journal of Sex Research*.[43] Perhaps the popularity of MILF porn implies that as women become more sexually empowered, men are seeking to share in the excitement and attraction of this movement?

Or perhaps MILF porn's meteoric rise can be attributed not only to the sexual dominance that actresses in MILF porn express, but to the fact that they feel more real and accessible. In an interview with *Playboy Magazine* on the topic of "Why Do Guys Like MILFs?", psychologist David Ley proposed that women in MILF porn are popular because they "look more real, like (they) could live down the street".[44] Now I'm not exactly sure what type of MILF porn he's watching, because there are still plenty of 30-year-old size 2s with DD breasts, perfect hair and flawless skin playing the "MILFs". Still, perhaps in general, the women in MILF porn seem slightly more authentic than their 18-year-old porn star counterparts. In his interview, Ley comments that when it comes to fantasies, for some men it is more exciting and appealing to fantasize about a woman who resembles someone he could actually meet and potentially have sex with in real life.

Likewise, women's searches also include numerous taboos like step-dad and daughter, lesbian scissoring and two separate references to gang bangs. People often watch porn to learn about things they do not understand, like, "Where do all the dicks go in a gangbang?" Or, "How large are these alleged BBCs (Big Black Cocks)?" Or, "What are the sexiest positions to use in a threesome?" Even though porn is fantasy and not necessarily real (because thankfully real-life sex does not have to look good on video, only feel good!), sometimes watching it can satiate our curiosity or spur us on to learn more.[45]

Over one-quarter of college-age women in the US report having one or more lesbian experiences according to a recent poll.[46] It hardly a surprise then that many women enjoy and even prefer watching lesbian porn to heterosexual porn. Maybe it is because the men in heterosexual porn can be overly aggressive, or maybe it is because lesbian porn seems more authentic? There has even been a rise in lesbian erotica made by women, and/ or featuring "regular" girls, without the fake boobs and tons of makeup, or with alternative vibes like piercings, tattoos or goths. Furthermore, many women feel that forms of erotica produced, directed and starring women tend to feel safer, more accessible and more sensual.

Is Watching Pornography a Psychological Problem?

Viewing pornography or erotica remains as old as art, or even human culture itself. Still, politicians and governments just love getting involved in our sex lives, from telling women what to do with their bodies, to dictating what types of porn or erotica constitute as "too extreme". Indeed, it was not until the landmark US Supreme Court ruling on *Stanley v Georgia* in 1969 that possessing pornography (which was previously viewed as an "obscene" material) became legal. (Of course, we know that this does not relate to child pornography, which is totally illegal and fundamentally wrong to create and possess, because children and teens under the age of 18 in the US cannot give affirmative consent!)

Recently, at least in America, lawmakers are still trying to restrict the use of and access to legal pornography. For example, in late 2016 Virginia lawmakers attempted to implement greater restrictions on the viewing of porn, claiming it is a "public health hazard" and "addictive" although there is little, if any, clinical evidence to support such a claim. Besides, we know from going to the grocery store that just because a substance is highly addictive does not mean that the state is responsible for controlling or banning it. A quick look at the availability of proven, harmfully addictive substances like alcohol, cigarettes and sugar in every single town in the US makes it almost comical that a state would be more concerned about strengthening regulations for "porn addiction". It's almost like they are afraid of sex or something.

Many psychologists and psychotherapists currently tend to view pornography in terms of a public health issue rather than an addiction issue. In fact, some psychologists like David Ley and colleagues (2014) argue that porn addiction is not real (when compared with other addictions), and that the theory and research behind pornography addiction is "hindered by poor experimental designs, limited methodological rigor, and lack of model specifications".[47] Psychological research in this area has failed to show any empirical effects of the erectile dysfunction or brain rewiring allegedly caused by watching too much porn. However, a 2014 study showed a correlation between reduced grey matter in the brain and hours per week spent watching porn,[48] but this is not causation, meaning it is possible that people with less grey matter are naturally drawn to watching porn.[49] With such a small sample size in clinical settings, more research needs to be conducted to determine if watching porn is really the *cause* of sexually compulsive behaviour or merely a symptom of it.

As of now, the *Diagnostic Statistical Manual of Psychology* (DSM-V) does not support the diagnosis of pornography addiction, and hypersexuality more broadly, as a valid clinical illness, determining that "there is insufficient peer-reviewed evidence to establish the diagnostic criteria and descriptions needed to identify these behaviours as mental health disorders."[50] Yes, you may have heard of anecdotal cases of people who claim to be "addicted" to pornography or say they require it for their sexual arousal, but Brand and colleagues (2016) argue that pornography addiction is better described as part of a larger symptom of the addictive nature of the Internet, or as part of an "Internet-use disorder".[51]

As we know, the tendency to pathologize anything that goes against the sexual norms of society remains common, so perhaps it is no surprise that the lack of clinical validation has not stopped people from cashing in on the business of treating pornography addiction. In 2014 the acclaimed film *Don Jon*, about a young male addicted to porn, thrust the idea very much into the limelight. In the film, the hours that Jon spends watching porn make it harder for him to interact with real women, although contrarily, some research suggests that people who watch more porn may actually be having more sex! For example, according to a survey of 1,000 Americans from the IFOP Institute, the people who watched the most porn also had the most partners and the most sex during the past year.[52]

In the context of looking at pornography use from a public health perspective, if you are an informed adult, you get to make informed decisions about how you spend your time. So long as you are not causing harm to anyone else, you can choose to eat 1,000 cheeseburgers, drink a fifth of a bottle of whiskey or smoke an entire carton of cigarettes. You can also choose who to hook up with, and you can choose who to watch having sex, so long as everyone is a consenting adult. We are not powerless bystanders in our lives; in fact, being sex positive dictates that we are autonomous beings who make informed choices about our behaviours.

When it comes to pornography, we are being fed fantasy and entertainment, just like every other form of media we consume: Porn is here to sexually excite you, not to teach or educate you about real life. So long as you realize this, there is probably nothing wrong with watching porn. I enjoy watching porn alone or with my partners, and it can be fun and arousing. But I'm not here thinking that everything I see in porn is the truth or that I should be comparing myself to the actresses in the film (just like I don't watch Marvel's *Thor* expecting lightning to shoot out of my fingertips, either). Remember that pornography only highlights a very small range of genitalia and body types, so please stay woke enough see it for what it is: Mindless entertainment designed to turn you on.

Nearly every human feels sexually repressed in some small or large way, as we often grow up believing that our sexual feelings or desires are immoral, wrong or just plain weird. Yet, there really is no such thing as "too weird" for porn. If you imagine the weirdest sexual thing you can think of, the porn for it probably already exists! Porn offers a space to explore and engage in these secret, strange parts of us, without having to commit or put any real effort in to changing ourselves or our partners. We can take a little peek behind the curtain, dipping a toe in the water from the safety of our living room. If you feel that you are compulsively watching porn and cannot stop, or you feel that is damaging your life or relationships, or you are concerned that you cannot become aroused without it, then maybe it has become a problem for you to address, most notably by first taking a break and seeing how you feel.

Changing Porn, Changing Sex Lives

No matter how you feel about porn, it truly does offer something for everyone. Even our engagement with porn is evolving as we enter the exponential technical growth of the *VR* (virtual reality) revolution. It's true that you currently need a headset and/or other gear to fully immerse yourself in VR porn, but according to PornHub, VR is becoming increasingly popular, with views rising exponentially since it was introduced in 2016. Piper Jaffray research analyst Travis Jakel predicts that in 2020, the VR porn industry will be worth over $1 billion, making it the third most important driver of VR tech development behind video games and movies.[53] Perhaps it is no surprise then that in 2018, *Fortnite* (a video game) was the fastest growing search term on PornHub in 2018 (and yes, before you ask, a quick search will reveal a massive new genre of porn that resembles the most popular video games).

In the near future we may expect blended sexual environments to become commonplace, which will bring holographic 3D representations of adult performers directly into our actual space. Imagine features like integrated remote sex devices, binaural sound and 360 degree viewing angles. People may soon be integrating their VR porn usage with haptic sex toys that mimic the content of the porn, making the experience feel even more real. Soon, our physical biology will also become augmented in our use of sexual entertainment. In a 2016 interview, futurist Ian Pearson proposed that by 2030, we will have VR contact lenses inserted directly into our eyes projecting high resolution graphics onto the retina, without even noticing we are wearing them.[54] Pearson also predicts that these lenses will pair with "active skin" – a technology linking sex toys and sexual stimuli from pornography directly to the nervous system. Thus, as we browse porn in the future, our brains may actually *experience* lifelike neurological stimulations of all five senses almost identical to the real thing. Whether this will feel like a huge turn-on or an unnatural assault to the senses remains to be seen, but it does beg the question, with so many technological innovations, will we even need a real human to have sex with in the near future?

Sex, Love and Relationships with Virtual Entities, Dolls and Robots

What makes porn unique is that it has always been a completely simulated experience. Even with VR porn, your favourite porn star will not jump through the screen at the end to make you climax, no matter real holograms could feel in the future. Sure, people have tried to get around this with technology that others can control such as webcams where the viewers can pay to activate the dildos or sybians (a type of vibrator resembling sexual furniture that you can ride) and so on (these streaming cam sites are becoming increasingly popular). But still, for most of us laypeople there will always been a sharp dividing line between the porn stars we enjoy watching on screen, and the people in our living rooms watching (or hopefully helping) us get excited.

But what if we really could make our fantasies come true, right in our own living rooms? Not through paying for escorts or hiring porn stars for sex, or even through buying realistic sex dolls or incredibly versatile sex toys. What if it was possible to create a lifelike sex doll of your favourite porn star who also was engineered specifically just to please you? Perhaps it is no surprise that as technology pushes the limits of what is possible, "sexbots" are shaping up to be one of our greatest new sex trends – and it has been predicted that by 2033, adult film actors will be selling robotic replicas of themselves designed exclusively for sex.[55]

Technically, sexbots already exist: Abyss Creations launched "Harmony AI" animatronic sex dolls in 2018, as well as robotic "heads" (yes, really) that can be attached to existing inanimate sex dolls to give them lifelike qualities including facial movement, conversation and personalities. Their dolls, called "*Realdolls*", essentially function as sexbots made from silicon and software with personalities that can be customized by owners across traits including kindness, shyness, naïveté, intellectualism, wit and sensuality. The creators of the dolls have already launched the Harmony virtual girlfriend app to give thousands of regular users the chance to see how it feels to be in an emotional relationship with a virtual being created solely to please them. Patrons can customize the bodies and personalities of virtual online girlfriends, including everything from skin tone, specific genitalia, hairstyle and colour, piercings and so on. Users can also tailor specific beauty features like hair, lip and nail colours. Between glass eyeballs and pubic hair made from alpaca fur, no expense is being spared! And for women out there, don't worry, even though most sex dolls are made with heterosexual men in mind, companies like Abyss are working to create male robotic dolls as well. Currently, male dolls account for about 10 per cent of their sales and have fewer customizable options, although popularity is rising thanks to headlines touting male sex dolls with "unstoppable bionic penises" coming soon![56]

If this entire topic creeps you out even a little bit, rest assured you are not alone. A spokesman for Abyss even says that while "most users like the idea of a woman created to serve them, others notice something missing". Hmmm … I wonder what could possibly be missing?[57] The videos of assembly lines constructing these dolls seem creepy to say the least, and while actual sales figures are hard to pin down, the dolls themselves seem to be pretty popular. (There are entire fandom subcultures of people who call themselves "IDollators", for example.) Despite the apparent popularity of sex dolls, manufacturers stress that they seek to make the dolls imperfect and not too human-like because they don't want to freak people out – this is related to a psychological prediction known as the *Uncanny Valley*.[58]

Sexbots remain poised to revolutionize not only interpersonal sex, but also the sex industry as we know it. Already in Spain, an existing sex-doll brothel featuring Lumidolls says it hopes to become "fully AI" soon, transitioning into a fully robotic sex holiday resort (Hello, Westworld!). Recently, an Austrian brothel reported that its most popular prostitute is now a sex doll named Fanny, allegedly more popular than the human women who are employed there.[59] Erica, a Japanese engineered sex robot, was just cast as a TV presenter in Japan. Indeed, in his report on "The Future of Sex", British futurist Ian Pearson envisions "a future in which robotic brothels and strip clubs with computer-controlled dancers are normal".[60]

Meanwhile, in November 2017, Saudi Arabia announced that it had granted full citizenship to an AI robot named Sophia. The irony is not lost that in a country where women do not have equal rights, Sophia does not have to wear a hijab and may even have more rights than the actual human women who live in Saudi Arabia. I just wonder if Sophia will ever get slut shamed on the Internet for wearing too much makeup or a low-cut blouse? Or stoned for appearing too promiscuous?

If you think that the idea of fully automated sexbots is not going to happen in our lifetimes, unless you're already old AF, you are probably wrong. Buried in a monster report on AI by the Pew Research Center is a prediction that by 2025, sex robots will be "commonplace".[61] As with all new technologies, a significant cost-based barrier to entry exists: The heads of the AI dolls alone cost upwards of $10,000, with full models costing as much as $50,000 for extremely customized versions like aliens or replicas of living people (which most companies promise they will not make without that person's consent). Currently, non-AI silicone sex dolls in the higher part of the market retail for about $5,000 each without automation. While sexbots and sex dolls are expensive now, like all technology, the price will inevitably drop low enough that the barrier to entry will begin to dissipate. Remember that flat screen that cost $5,000 in 2005? You could probably swoop it for $300 right now at Best Buy.

A 2017 UK study showed that of 263 heterosexual men surveyed, more than 40 per cent said they would consider purchasing a sex robot now or in the next five years.[62] Since the sexbot market is targeted overwhelmingly at men at present, a world where this many men have sexbots and/or robot girlfriends might force us to redefine what a "relationship" truly means. *The Future of Sex Report* (2016) predicts that by 2045, 1 in 10 young adults will have had sex with a humanoid robot, and this could be even higher if the technology develops quickly enough. But what if I told you that communities filled with thousands of men who have chosen sex dolls to be their wives and girlfriends already exist?[63]

Well, it's true. Life imitates art and art imitates life, and movies like *Lars and the Real Girl, Her* and *Blade Runner 2049* are seeming less like fiction and more like potential (albeit quirky) portals into relationships of the future. For many of the men on *The Doll Forum*, an online community of over 18,000 members, sex dolls represent a form of companionship with a woman on whom they can truly rely. Yes, the irony is real that for many men, the only woman they can rely upon is an inanimate one. But then again, many of the users report social anxiety about relating to women, in addition to negative past experiences in their relationships and other forms of childhood trauma that inhibit comfortable human to human relationships.

In a 2015 *Vice* exposé on IDollators, the overwhelming theme among doll lovers interviewed was "using dolls to replicate human presence". While they might look like creepy dead-eyed hunks of silicone to some, for the people in this community, the dolls represent not only a sex aid, but also an antidote to loneliness. One member explains that "it's like when a husband has his wife and kids come home, you know, I have that; I have someone at home." Another user says he thinks of his two dolls not as sex objects, but as surrogate adult daughters. He tells *Vice*, "I would like to have a human companion, but I find dating too stressful. I'm impotent with prostate issues, and if I marry, I'll lose retirement benefits – telling that to a real woman won't go down well."[64]

How the Technosexual Revolution is Redefining "Relationships"

Although sex dolls offer a physical presence that creates a comforting feeling for many of their lovers, for others out there, the psychological and emotional space matters even more. While ten years ago, the idea of "virtual girlfriends" was limited to video games and strangers in online chatrooms, there is now a plethora of apps used by millions of people as *dating simulators*. A quick search will show you top ten rankings of these, including *Naughty Girlfriend*, *Dream Girlfriend* and *My Virtual Girlfriend*. At the time of writing, *My Virtual Girlfriend*, the number one rated dating simulation app, has more than one million downloads on the Google Play Store. And so does *My Virtual Boyfriend*.

Just let that sink in for a moment. Who are these millions of people experimenting with virtual girlfriends and boyfriends? Are they all creepy socially awkward nerds tucked away in high-rise apartment buildings in Japan? Are they young insecure boys and girls with little to no experience with dating? Are they just too busy for an actual partner but still seek the love and attention of text messages and chats? Or do they find it more enjoyable to interact with a virtual person created solely for their entertainment, whose needs don't really matter? We honestly don't know, but there are probably many different reasons why people would use a dating simulator (maybe you are one of them?). Although it is tempting to assume that people who use these apps lack social skills and empathy, or have high levels of narcissism, nobody knows for sure why people are using these simulators (although I believe that loneliness is probably the underlying motivator).

The increasing popularity of virtual partners begs the question, will two people even be required for a relationship to exist in the future? The emotional ramifications of relationships with "fake" or synthetic partners are far-reaching, potentially redefining everything we think we know about romantic relationships and their functions. Social psychology is the study of people's impacts upon others, real or imagined. And it seems that in our near future, the "imagined" ones are poised to take centre stage. Movies like Spike Jonze's brilliant *Her* (2013) and Denis Villeneuve's *Blade Runner 2049* (2017) serve as allegories for the inevitable: People can and will fall in love with their virtual/holographic partners. Several futurists, such as David Levy in *Love and Sex with Robots* (2009), have predicted that in the next 20 to 30 years, we will be marrying our robots, and this will be regarded as a valid expression of our feelings of love and sexual desire. Ian Pearson also predicts that by 2050, human–robot sex will overtake human–human sex.[65]

Perhaps we can blame the Internet for opening the door to one-sided anonymous relationships, as the AOL chatrooms of the late 1990s enabled many people to build online romances with people they might have never met in person. Is it really that much of a stretch to find the same connection with an app or a doll, even if we know there isn't a living a breathing person behind it? Think about how dating apps like Tinder, OkCupid and Grindr have permanently altered the face of dating as we know it (more on this in chapter 9). Five years ago, people were looking for love on Craigslist, ten years ago it was still a little taboo to send dick pics, and 15 years ago everyone was getting down with Myspace hookups. Before that, we actually had to venture out and learn to chat up someone in real life if we wanted to get it on! Now we just swipe right … It seems like virtual partners and sex robots could serve as natural progressions of our desires to meet our sexual needs using technology, and to do so in a quick, efficient way.

For now, people who love their sex dolls are still very much on the fringe, but in retrospect they could be hailed as visionaries who rewrote the story about love and sex. The term *digisexual* is already being proposed as a stigma-free alternative sexual identity for people whose sexual desires are satisfied by the virtual, digital and/or online world. According to an article published in the *Journal of Sexual and Relationship Therapy* (2017), radical new sexual technologies mean that we can expect a rise of people who identify as digisexual, requiring psychologists to develop a new framework for understanding the social, legal and ethical implications of addressing a new generation of potential clients.[66] If statistics are accurate that 40 per cent of men may choose to purchase a sexbot, will the doll lovers of the future represent a marginalized minority, or will they pave the way for the mainstream to follow? Only time will tell.

The Debate Over Human–Robot Relationships

Whether you're excited or grossed out about our sexbot future, there are people out there who agree with you. The debates for and against sexbots are somewhat similar to those surrounding pornography. One side of the debate argues that sexbots could benefit people, particularly but not exclusively men who struggle with relational skills like communication and emotional attachment, potentially enriching their lives psychologically and emotionally. Sex robots could offer future opportunities to serve in therapeutic, as well as educational and advisory, contexts. In addition to providing immersive sex education, technological automations in sexuality could also lead to "robotic sex gurus" who become the ultimate lovers, able to learn and adapt their sexual skills to train humans to become better lovers.

The other side still puts forth a compelling argument that these sexbots objectify women and erode existing relationships between people, as they teach people to fall in love with non-human beings who do not have needs or feelings to be considered. While sex robots are theoretically always horny (ha!), some have argued adding a "resist" setting would help them be truer to real life. Others might argue that the Hitachi Magic Wand, a girl's best friend (when it comes to vibrators) and one of the greatest technological developments to aid women's orgasms, is also rather ... robotic! Can sex positive people really draw the line between the morally "right" and "wrong" sexual technologies!? It seems to go against the idea of people having the autonomy and freedom to express their sexuality as they choose.

It might be hard for some people to fathom the implications of a world inhabited by people and their robotic sex partners. I think back to the innocent joys of my Internet- and computer-free childhood, a lifetime which has been spent half without and half with easy access to the Internet (first email at 14, my first cellphone at 18, and so on). If those of us born between 1977 and 1983 are called "*Xennials*" – a sub generation of those who grew up without technology but who have spent at least half their lives now with technology – I wonder if there will be another generation like this in the future (maybe called the "*robo-ennials?*") who spent half their lives without robots and half of their lives living with them?

A Sex Positive Perspective

On a more basic psychological and emotional level, if people experience therapeutic benefits from having a virtual partner or from loving sex dolls, or if the mere imagined or implied presence of "something" at home makes them feel happy, more complete and less lonely, then can an outsider judge their behaviours as right or wrong? Clinically, it is unclear if such digisexual behaviour would qualify as a sexual dysfunction, if the person's needs are being met and no harm is being done to themselves or others. Being sex positive, we must once again avoid the urge to pathologize non-normative sexual behaviours and remain open minded to multiple permutations and evolutions of human sexuality.

Humans possess an innate desire to feel loved and accepted, and clearly, as technology develops, the way that humans set benchmarks for these needs and seek to satiate them must necessarily evolve. Spiritually, emotionally and psychologically, will relationships with automatons/cyborgs/robots or holograms be as fulfilling as relationships with breathing, real-life humans? It would not be possible to make broad sweeping generalizations here, because we simply do not know. As globalization arguably continues to create a more physically isolated world, can we really blame those who are lonely and bored for seeking some semblance of connection? When it was revealed that a Chinese chatbot named "*Xiaoice*", spoken to by 89 million people, had been told "I love you" nearly 20 million times, should we question whether it made people feel good to say "I love you", or should we be questioning whether these people could be saying it to a flesh-and-blood human?[67]

Humans have always sought new and innovative ways to meet their sexual and psychological needs. While the concept of a virtual girlfriend or boyfriend might not be right for me at this moment, I also did not grow up with a tablet strapped to my hands and a Facebook page created by my parents before I was even born, so who am I to judge someone else's desires or relationship choices? Growing up so intertwined with technology makes us increasingly more likely to accept and engage in a romantic relationship with machines or non-human entities. We simply cannot predict how far this trend will extend, but one thing is for sure: It is already happening.

In hindsight, we can see clearly how a multitude of technological inventions have been utilized to benefit people's sex lives. Sex swings, sex cushions, Viagra, strap-ons, dildos of all kinds, pocket pussies and rabbit vibes are all examples of the technosexual revolution where humans have allowed machines or innovations into the bedroom to enhance our sexual pleasure and fulfilment. New sex toys are even being developed to help women cope with losing their pelvic floor after childbirth or menopause, as well as helping survivors of sexual trauma feel comfortable with being touched again. Sex-toy innovations designed to benefit survivors of sexual assault include a horse-hair brush for exploring touch and tickling, a special mirror designed to help women get a better view of their vulvas, a bean-shaped sensor that lights up if the user is breathing too fast (encouraging them to slow down and relax), a pelvic device that vibrates when the muscles of the vagina become too tense, as well as a variety of unassuming, non-phallic clitoral vibrators. And while I've heard anecdotal arguments about women who lose clitoral sensitivity from overuse of vibrators, I can't say I know too many women who have complained about having access to a Magic Wand when they wanted one. (We will talk more in chapter 5 about sex toys, orgasms and new innovations designed to close the orgasm gap during vaginal penetrative sex!)

From a sex positive perspective, we must remain open to the idea that sex with virtual partners may become integrated into our sexual development in the future. In *The Future of Sex Report*, Dawson and Owsianik predict that by 2028, over one-quarter of all sexually active adults will have had a long-distance sexual experience.[68] Many of us are already sexting, camming and DM'ing (direct messaging) our partners today. If humans can gain the psychological sense of love and inclusion, as well as sexual gratification, from merely the implied existence of other humans, can they not also experience it with autonomic identities? This certainly seems likely.

Transhumanistic Sexual Bio-Hacking
We should also wonder how the technosexual revolution redefines love and sex even for people who opt out of having their own personal sex robot or virtual girlfriend. Will real-life humans be getting any action at all, having to compete with realistic robots whose sole function persists in providing sexual satisfaction to others? Ian Pearson (2016) argues that yes, even though human–robot sex will become more common, humans will still have sex with other humans, and that by 2050 the same

technology that facilitates human–robot sex will also be used to enhance human–human sex. Notably, he predicts we will be able to link our brains and nervous systems together, thus feeling our partner's pleasures as if they were our own. He elaborates that:

> By 2050, if your partner is fully connected to you and you can directly feel the sensations that you're generating in your partner, it will make you a better lover as well. You will know that your partner's enjoying it because you'll be able to feel they're enjoying it. So, you'll be able to get really close to the other person, much closer than you can today, so the technology isn't just about sterilizing these relationships, it's about making them deeper ... I think the fact that the same technology allows you to have closer relationships with human beings tends to get left aside, when I think that it's just as important ... You'll be able to be one with your partner in a way that you just can't today.[69]

Not to be outdone by robots, the technosexual revolution promises that humans will seek to harness the same sexual technologies used by AI sexbots to augment our own sexual pleasure and performance. Dawson and Owsianik (2016) predict that biohackers will attempt to turn themselves into sexual cyborgs by manipulating their physical form and biology. In this vision of the future, "sci-fi sex fantasies will spring into life as people can enhance their biology and merge with machines to become superhuman sex idols."[70] From this transhumanistic perspective, humans are constantly seeking to enhance ourselves to transcend the limits of our biology, sometimes to extremes. Biohacker Richard Lee (2017) has proposed the Lovetron 9000, a motorized device implanted above the male pubic bone that essentially turns a man into a human vibrator. He already has a working prototype and has partnered with Ascendance Biomedical to develop it.[71] Lee also plans a sexual biohacking device for women that will be implanted in the labia and squeeze the clitoris via two electromagnets on either side.

Futurists have consistently painted a picture of a world where humans will essentially become sexual cyborgs, using a range of advanced surgical techniques, gene editing, lab-grown genital implants and/or tissue engineering to enhance and customize our sexual bodies. But can we predict how this will impact our sex lives and identities? Is biohacking productive for those of us pursuing sex positive lives, or just a necessary evil of humanity's developmental trajectory?

The Human Cost of Redefining Love

Psychologically, the changing nature of love reflects one of the largest confounds of burgeoning human–machine relationships. Anyone who has been in love, or been in a relationship, understands how potentially messy and difficult the experience of human love can feel. In fact, one of the predominant features of human–human love is the level of sacrifice and compromise required in nearly all types of loving and romantic relationships. This is perhaps why some of the most beloved art, music and film that has emerged from human culture, especially in our generation and those before us, reflects the themes of unrequited or lost love, and of the incredible difficulties we must endure as part of our commitment to human relationships. There is a melancholic sorrow in the way that we fight to love and to connect with each other, and perhaps part of what makes falling in love so beautiful and alluring is that we know we will make sacrifices: We accept that by opening our hearts we have chosen to embark on a challenging and potentially painful or destructive journey. For many of us, maybe the risk itself can become the greatest turn-on? (Eat your heart out Freud!)

If the rawest essence of human relationships becomes embodied by the sacrifices that we endure for love, what does this mean for love in the technosexual age? Will romantic love itself begin to lose the qualities with which it has become so heavily endowed, and take on a different significance altogether? Surely falling in love with a machine programmed to please and pander to your every whim negates some of the essential qualities that have become equated with our conception of romantic love? I sometimes sit back and wonder if my generation or the one directly following us (Generation-Z) might be the very last to experience human romantic love in its rawest, most intense form, where nothing is certain and making things work can feel so confusing and difficult. Falling in love with your own personal sexbot or virtual partner would heavily mitigate the risk and rewards of love, removing the suffering and perhaps also the exaltation, that comes from relationships. Is it still love if you know you are safe, if you know you cannot be hurt, if you know you are in control, and if you know your partner's needs don't matter if they can be shut off with the switch of a button?

Some people see this new conception of love as a benefit and argue that non-human sex partners could prove their worth to humanity by offering us the opportunity to remove the potential human suffering that comes with falling in love. They are baiting us into a world without heartbreak and giving us power over the one thing over which we humans have never had control: The feelings and needs of our partners. While there is something to be said for building a world where relationships are less difficult and less painful, I would counter that in doing so, we would be inadvertently deleting the very aspect that makes love human: Its messiness, and our lack of ability to control it. Will a person who grows up in a world of customized, machine-made lovers really ever know what heartbreak feels like? Will they be able to dive to the same emotional depths, and to create the same art fuelled by romantic pain, that we have?

In my personal experience, the suffering and sacrifices I have made for love have become a huge part of my own humanity and remain integral to my personal growth. Removing that from the equation sounds positively alien to me, as I struggle to connect with the person I might be if I had never known these challenges. Of course, anyone in the throes of heartbreak might say they wish they never had to feel such pain, but even the worst breakup can serve us up a pile of sludge with a diamond underneath the surface just waiting to be uncovered and polished. As we push further into the technosexual revolution, my hope is that we will not be willing to let go of the very elements that make our love human. People with sex positive attitudes must keep in mind the deep and inherent differences between sex and love, which are subjectively defined by each person, as well as the ever-blurring boundaries between humans and machines. I hope that we can create virtual and robotic partners that are not completely submissive to humans, but that can at least mimic the elements of human relationships that challenge us and help us grow into the best sex positive people we can become. But in order to do that, we must first fully understand our own changing attitudes and identities and figure out how to work through the individual challenges posed by the shifting narrative about love and sex.

PART TWO

REDEFINING OURSELVES

CHAPTER 4

SEX AS A SPIRITUAL EXPERIENCE

The transforming social landscape of love and sex indicates some deeper changes happening within us, with respect to our own identities. Many people naturally assume that our bodies and physical health (including our sexual health!) are somehow separate from our mind and spirit, including our emotional, mental and spiritual health. We are taught that humans possess innate mating-based sex drives that dominate our desires and behaviours, over which we have very little control. We know that our hormones contribute to our sexual development, but we have barely begun to understand the psychology of how our neurochemistry paired with fuel we put into our bodies can affect the relationship between these hormones and our emotional states. Over the past few centuries, human sexuality has been treated like a physiological and biological formula. Only recently have we begun to factor into the equation how our consciousness and sexual energies interact with our physical experiences to paint a complete picture of our sexualities.

The push for a mind-body-spirit approach to sexuality has become quite important to many of us. A holistic approach makes sense when we consider how sexuality is something that exists at the very core of each of our beings. We use our sexuality, through intercourse and procreation, to connect to the divine energies out in the universe and pull them into our physical bodies to give them life. Whether you think that sounds like BS or not, when we break it down to the core of the matter, sex creates life. Nothing else but sex can do that. Literally nothing. (Yet!) We can harness our sexual energies as a positive creative force in our lives, not only through having intercourse, but also through connecting more deeply to our sexual energies and using them to build intimacy and trust with other people.

Thanks to modern-day philosophers, life coaches, scientists and healers like Ekhart Tolle, Dr Bruce Lipton, Sara Beak, Louise Hay, Dr Joe Dispenza, Gabrielle Bernstein and many more, we are beginning to cut through the isolation created by globalization and technology as we seek to redefine our humanity and sense of self. We are looking for meaning not only outside of ourselves, but also *within* ourselves. We are currently in the midst of what I can only call a *neo-spiritual revolution* focused on integrating mind, body and spirit while pursuing esoteric, ancient, neo-shamanic, energetic or dare I say "spiritual" methods for reconnecting to our truest essences, breaking through the conditioning of a sick society and returning to the deep knowledge that lies within us about who we are and what we came here to do.

Think about it: Yoga, an ancient meditative practice that integrates body, mind and spirit, has become one of the most popular approaches to relaxation and fitness across the world. The yoga industry itself has grown exponentially over the past ten years, and is currently estimated to be worth about $16 billion annually in the US and over $80 billion globally.[72] Sure, we could argue that the yoga that we practise in the West differs tremendously from traditional yoga, but when it comes down to it, we are still pursuing healing, relaxation and joy by participating in these ancient traditions and reaping the benefits – even in our sex lives! Yoga helps us reduce anxiety, lower our stress hormone levels and helps us reconnect (the word "yoga" translates to "yoke", as in, yoking us back into our bodies). Studies have shown that regular yoga practice improves multiple levels of sexual functioning in women (including desire, arousal, lubrication, orgasm, satisfaction and pain) as well as enhancing desire, intercourse satisfaction, performance, confidence, partner synchronization, erection, ejaculatory control, and orgasm in men.[73] Maybe that's why we've been trading our party holidays for yoga retreats in lush tropical climates like Costa Rica and Bali.

Perhaps we crave yoga because we are consistently diagnosed as the *most anxious generation ever* and we know we need to find a way to decompress. Statistics continue to show how millennials have higher incidences of depression, anxiety and suicidal ideation than all previous generations, and new findings suggest that we can blame this on our increased levels of perfectionism.[74] Our mental health is suffering because we put so much pressure on ourselves to excel across nearly every area of life, an affliction that psychologists call *multidimensional perfectionism*. Why is this happening to us? In part, this is because our society now places a greater emphasis on meritocracy, competitiveness, educational attainment and individualism than ever before. We have the pushiest, most anxious parents ever. And social media is constantly here to remind us of all the things we don't have, ramping up our competitiveness and our desires to succeed in the eyes of the world. Traditional medicine and psychiatry attempt to help us cope by prescribing combination stimulants like amphetamine/dextroamphetamine to rev us up so we can get everything done, paired with downers like alprazolam so that we can calm down and sleep. Many mental health professionals (myself included) feel that this pharmaceutical "speed ball" might do more harm than good for some of us in the long term.

Our unparalleled anxiety, matched with the lack of efficacy of traditional treatments, may explain why we are driving the marketplace for functional medicine solutions, alternative therapies and integrative health care. We are even rediscovering and tweaking esoteric and ancient healing modalities in a desperate push to find peace in a chaotic, pressure-filled world. We seek therapies that will actually *work* to treat the causes of our issues, not just the symptoms. Consider the growing popularity of herbal healing, essential oil therapies, acupuncture, Traditional Chinese Medicine, cupping, Ayurveda, Kambo frog medicine, reflexology and so on. Even the field of psychology is witnessing unprecedented advances in alternative therapies, from art healing, to sound healing, to somatic therapies, to psychedelic therapy. For example, ketamine (an anaesthetic typically used on animals and vulnerable populations which has maintained a psychedelic "club drug" reputation for many years) is not only legal when prescribed by a psychologist in some states in the US, but is being hailed as *the* breakthrough in psychiatric treatment for depression in the 21st century.

What an intense time to be alive! We know we are anxious and depressed, but we are actively searching for real, authentic answers that actually make us feel healthier and more complete, rather than papering over the cracks so that we can keep pushing forward. Rediscovering and reconnecting our minds, bodies and spirits remains paramount to our wellness. Whether we realize it or not, and even with the many obstacles we face, many of us are beating a path to a healthy, thriving and connected version of ourselves. Sure, some of us take many detours to get there (hey, it's part of the healing process!) but the answer is still the same: As we redefine the core attitudes that shape our lives, we must also grow and evolve ourselves. Sexuality plays an important role here because our sexual energy represents our life-giving, connected, creative qualities. I believe that if we want to help reduce our anxiety and depression, we must embrace our holistic sexuality to build meaning in our lives and forge deeper connections with each other. We are beginning to reclaim sexuality as an energetic or spiritual experience because it is important for our individual and collective growth, bringing us back to what it means to be truly human. This helps us shred the layers of social conditioning to build upon the ancient wisdom of the past to create a new future that truly serves us.

You might be asking: Dr Kelly, you are a scientist, do you really believe in all this woo-loo-shanti stuff?

Sex and Energy: My Story

Yes, I do. Ok maybe not in everything, but there are definitely components of the connection between energy and the sexual body that I do believe in. And I'm going to tell you why.

It stems from my personal experiences with phenomena that I cannot explain using science or logic. Remember my story about my traumatic uterus surgeries and near-death experience? What I haven't told you yet is what happened the day I went into surgery. As I was being wheeled into the operating theatre and starting to lose consciousness, I suddenly shot awake, grabbed the surgeon by both hands and asserted, "You have my consent to do a full hysterectomy!" Taken aback, she explained to me for the thousandth time that I didn't need a full hysterectomy, I just needed a myomectomy to remove two tumours, and that I'd keep the rest of my uterus (when you are a 30-year-old woman with no children, doctors are unbelievably twitchy about performing a hysterectomy unless you're near death – which I happened to be, but even *still* they didn't want to do it). I said it again, that I consented to a hysterectomy, and then I passed out from the anaesthesia.

Eight hours later, I woke up in the recovery room from what should have been a two-hour surgery. The surgeon was there, and she told me that I was in fact *correct* – I did need a full hysterectomy. In spite of multiple MRIs and ultrasounds performed at some of the top hospitals in the country, my uterus did not contain two tumours like they thought, but *over two thousand*. She said that in fifteen years of uterine surgery she had never seen a uterus so warped. It was the size of a seven-month pregnancy! They tried to remove as many tumours as possible, but as I began to haemorrhage, they had no choice but to perform the full hysterectomy, which, by some higher power or deep knowledge inside of myself, I knew was going to happen.

The intuition that alerted me to the true needs of my body from an anaesthetized, near-comatose state would be enough to prove to myself that on some level, we have a deeper energetic connection between our minds and sexual bodies than we realize. But my story doesn't end there. No, as the surgeon was describing my uterus, she told me that my uterus "looked like a bunch of grapes". Despite being under a heavy dose of post-surgery opioids, the hairs on my entire body stood up and I felt like my heart was going to stop beating right there in my chest. Why?

Remember how I told you that my partner used to do Reiki on me, holding his hands over my body when I was writhing in agony from the pain of the tumours? We would call them his "energy hands" because through using his Reiki techniques, he could sometimes "see" inside of people's bodies, send healing light energy to clear out blockages. He had done this for hundreds of people in medical environments during his training. And while the energy hands did give me some relief from the pain, I never did know if it was a placebo or the actual Reiki really doing the work. Time and time again, and we're talking years before any of the scans or the surgeries, he would say to me, "Babe, your uterus looks like a bunch of grapes."

When I heard those words come out of my surgeon's mouth, I didn't know whether to laugh, cry, scream, punch her in the face, or pass out. It triggered a rush of emotions that to this very day I have never felt again. I locked eyes with my partner across the room and mouthed "grapes" to him, to make sure I wasn't imagining things or hallucinating having just come out of surgery. But it was real. His hands, using energy work techniques, were better predictors of the state of my sex organs than multiple MRI machines, ultrasounds and doctors. Holy crap!

Looking back now, I sometimes wonder if I had to go through this entire experience just to grab that little gold nugget at end of the rainbow which offered me a sense of irrefutable proof that the sexual energy is *real,* but when it becomes blocked, it can manifest in the body as tumours, illness or other types of illness. The notion of repressed emotional pain leading to physical symptoms is certainly nothing new, as Louise Hay pioneered many of these ideas during the New Age movement.[75] Is it really so much of a stretch that energetic blockages could have the same impact upon the body? Certainly, one of the core philosophies of Reiki healing involves clearing energetic blockages to reduce physical symptoms and increase overall wellbeing. It makes sense that this was the practice my partner used when he diagnosed the "bunch of grapes" in my uterus. In the case of my sex organs, it seemed especially profound that my partner who I loved so dearly was the only person amidst dozens of specialists who was actually right about what was going on inside of me. Maybe it was because he was using energetic techniques to address what was fundamentally created by repressed energies? Perhaps you have a similar story? Or maybe you think I'm just making this up. But I promise you, it's true. And while you don't have to be "spiritual" to believe that this could happen, it certainly does help.

Spiritual, Not Necessarily Religious

I guess you could say that the near-death experience I had gave me a sense of spirituality or a belief in something "more" than just our observable, physical reality. This is a fairly common experience. When people go through intense trauma, if they survive, they tend to come out of it with a sense of purpose or faith in a higher power. But what was interesting for me (and has been the case with many people I've spoken with about this topic), the higher power isn't the literal God as we know it from monotheistic religions, nor is it the Hindu gods or the Buddha. (FYI, I'm still pretty agnostic when it comes to the existence of a literal "God".) No, the faith I feel has more to do with a belief in the subtle energies that we cannot see but that have always been there, working behind the scenes to connect us more deeply to ourselves and each other. We can call this the universal quantum field, the spirit energy, the divine, love frequency, and a host of other names. We are connected to it and always influencing it. This is not a religious experience; it is a spiritual one.

The difference? Religion is all about a belief in the principles of an organized system of faith and worship and its teachings. Spirituality on the other hand refers to an individual's connection with "the divine", which manifests as an individual process of beliefs and practices that evolves over time. You've probably heard the phrase, "religion is for people afraid going to hell, and spirituality is for people who have already been there." People in new age circles have coined the term *SBNR* (Spiritual But Not Religious) to reflect their rejection of the organized structure of religion in favour of the pursuit of their individual mind-body-spirit connections One of the key philosophical distinctions between millennials and all previous generations is that by most measures, we are the least "religious" generation ever. A 2018 Pew Research Center poll found that while two-thirds of US adults over 50 believe in "God", less than half of those under 30 agree. They also found in 2015 that 40 per cent of millennials say that "religion is very important" compared with nearly 60 per cent of baby boomers and 72 per cent of the greatest generation (our grandparents).[76] But we are not just faithless heathens (well, some of us are and that's ok, ha!).

A 2018 joint US–UK study commissioned by Vice Media in partnership with the Insight Strategy Group found that more than 80 per cent of millennials and Gen-Z "had a sense of spirituality and believed in a higher cosmic power" with an additional 3 out of 4 saying that they did not want to impose any religion on their children.[77] Seven out of ten also said that they actively search for spirituality in their lives. The take-home message of the report? "Millennials and Gen-Z have all but rejected organized religion. They are extremely spiritual, but they have found a myriad of other ways to express and nurture that spirituality outside of religion." So, what stimulates our souls and gives us a sense of spirituality? According to respondents, the number one answer was listening to music, attending concerts and music festivals, followed by engaging in self-care, talking to friends, going for hikes and walks and creating art or writing. Organized religion (such as attending church services) was all the way down at number 18 on the list. Some older adults might herald this as the "breakdown of society" and we might agree, but not for the same reasons.

The Vice survey suggests that our spirituality is broadly undefined and can take on many non-traditional forms. I've worked extensively on the transformational festival circuit (at events like Sonic Bloom and Lucidity) doing talks and workshops about sexuality, and I can attest that these are often highly spiritual experiences for people. Something about the music, healthy food, yoga, psychedelics and sense of community triggers people to reveal deeper parts of themselves, connecting back to the tribal gatherings of our ancient human past. Paganism and Wicca have made huge comebacks too, offering feelings of empowerment and sisterhood/brotherhood to those who might have felt like they were on the fringe a decade ago. The tarot card/mediumship/astrology/aura reading industry alone is valued at over $2 billion annually according to Market Watch.[78] It was a little shocking to read a 2014 survey showing that the majority of young adults in America now believe that astrology is at least "somewhat" scientific.[79] Yes, we are much more open-minded than previous generations, but are we becoming too open? Maybe our beliefs in astrology can be explained by self-fulfilling prophecy (as in, we believe in astrology, so it feels real to us) or maybe we are just looking for meaning in places that make sense to our lifestyles and identities.

When it comes to sexuality specifically, it has been incredible to see new traditions and rituals springing up that reflect some level of a spiritual connection and a desire to connect to our ancient pasts. For example, the study of sexual astrology (the matching of astrological signs for the purpose of successful relationships) has become increasingly mainstream. There are so many different topics I could discuss here, but for the sake of space I'll just mention a few that have attracted my attention.

Spiritual Sexuality Trends

"*Rent tent*" parties are sisterhood-focused gatherings of women that have been traditionally used to celebrate *menarche*, or a woman's first period. Also called "*first moon*" parties, they are designed to overcome period shaming and encourage women to embrace this necessary part of their divine feminine sides. These gatherings usually happen in a space with red candles, beads and clothing where the women hold hands, sing and say prayers or chants. Pagan or witchy by nature, these parties have extended beyond first period parties and in most US cities you can now find monthly gatherings where women of all ages come to together, usually on the full moon or new moon, to connect to their divine feminine energies. Oh, and to talk about their periods. I've even been to gatherings where women actually wipe small amounts of their menstrual blood on their bodies, stemming from a belief that the life-giving lining of the uterus is a powerful energetic force.

Spirit Pussy Trends

These include using yoni eggs, usually fashioned from rose quartz or jade, that a woman can insert into her vagina to help stimulate her sexual energy and improve her pelvic floor. By keeping these eggs in your vagina all day long, proponents claim that your Kegels will get much stronger, which will lead to better sex. In practice, it is harder than you might think to keep those eggs in there! A lot of women report them just slipping right out. Can a stone in your vagina really make you feel more sensual? Maybe. But medically, I'm not sure if it's a good idea to keep anything in your vagina all day long, even a tampon, because of the risk of bacteria and toxic shock syndrome. Yoni eggs made headline news after Gwyneth Paltrow's wellness company GOOP agreed to pay out over $145,000 to consumers who purchased their jade yoni eggs at $66 each. The company was fined for falsely claiming that the eggs could "balance hormones, regulate menstrual cycles, prevent uterine prolapse, and increase bladder control".[80] While the jury is still out on the actual efficacy of yoni eggs to balance your sexual "chi", their rise to stardom over the past few years shows just how much we like the idea of empowering our pussies with spiritual goodies and toys.

Another spiritual pussy trend that's been making waves across the natural health world thanks to multiple celebrity endorsements is the idea of *yoni steams*, which basically means sitting with your vagina over a steaming hot bath of herbs. Steaming has been attributed with health benefits ranging from reducing painful menstrual symptoms, to promoting fertility and reducing stress, although there really isn't any scientific research to back up these claims. Touted as an ancient practice to enhance female sexual wellness and detoxify the womb, you can purchase a blend of herbs for around $20 on Amazon that includes rosemary, mugwort, motherwort, yarrow, calendula, lavender and rose petals. Often the yoni steam experience is augmented with guided meditations to maximize its cleansing effects. I'm all for pussy wellness, but I've never tried this (probably because I don't have a womb anymore!). Still, it shows our desire to integrate our modern spirituality with ancient techniques for wellness. Another trend that made headlines after a Hollywood actress claimed to do it regularly is *pussy sun bathing*, where you lie outside and open up your legs and allow the sun's rays to energize and cleanse your vagina. Have you or anyone you know you tried yoni eggs/steams or pussy sun bathing? What do you think?

Orgasmic Meditation Workshops

These offer a cautionary tale of what happens when spiritual sexuality goes wrong. You might have read articles a couple of years ago about these types of workshops springing up all over the country. Imagine two people: one of them is sitting up and fully clothed (can be any gender), while the other is a woman who is lying down, naked from the waist down. The fully clothed person, who is wearing a protective glove, proceeds to stimulate the woman's clitoris for 15 minutes. No other sexual contact happens, no kissing, no touching, no foreplay and certainly no penetration. Just plain old clitoral stimulation. This is called "*OMing*" and it is trademarked by a company called

OneTaste that, in 2017, made over $12 million doing orgasmic meditation workshops and retreats.

The philosophy underlying orgasmic meditation reflects the conscious, spiritual liberation of women's orgasms, by separating orgasmic release from the context of a relationship and allowing women to completely let go in the moment with another person, without the needs, expectations and demands that are usually put on them by other people. (Hmm, this doesn't sound that different from sex with robots now, does it?) Despite being touted by celebrities like Khloe Kardashian and hosting retreats that cost as much as $36,000 to attend, in 2018 OneTaste ceased all in-person orgasmic meditation classes and retreats to focus on online education, after *Bloomberg Business Week* published a bombshell report on predatory sales and recruitment practices at the company.[81] From many insiders it sounds as though the atmosphere at the company became almost cult like, as "many of the former staffers and community members say OneTaste resembled a kind of prostitution ring – one that exploited trauma victims and others searching for healing."

Well, if the meteoric rise and fall of orgasmic meditation can teach us anything, it is that the idea of conscious sexuality can excite and motivate us, piquing our curiosity about how to help women orgasm more frequently (and as we will discuss in the next chapter, some women struggle to find that true orgasmic release). Theoretically, I appreciate the idea of helping women to release and focus more on their orgasms. But the fact that some members felt that this practice became coercive or took advantage of the power dynamics involved is worrying to say the least. An upsetting part of the neo-spiritual movement materializes when gurus or mentors abuse their power and take advantage of their "disciples". Be wary. Consider the case of Bikram Choudhury (founder of the immensely popular Bikram yoga), who was accused of sexual assault by more than a dozen of his female students and colleagues and fled the US in 2017 after a warrant was issued for his arrest, for refusing to pay in a fraud judgement against him.[82] All people pursuing spiritual mentorship should remain vigilant when a guru or teacher uses sex as a method to establish dominance or control. Coercion is not sexy! And true spiritual growth can happen without anyone abusing their power or making anyone else feel obligated to do anything that makes them uncomfortable.

Psychedelic Sex Therapy
This is the use of psychedelic medicines like MDMA (3,4-methylenedioxymethamphetamine, also known as "molly" or ecstasy), psilocybin (derived from psychedelic mushrooms), ayahuasca (a psychedelic tea brewed from mimosa or acacia tree bark) or LSD (made from ergotamine fungus) for sexual healing. One could argue that the connection between psychedelic plant medicine and sexuality may go back thousands of years to human prehistory (if you agree with Terrence McKenna's evolutionary approach, that is) but even in modern history, the use of MDMA by psychotherapists and relationship therapists in the US during the late 1970s and early 1980s was well documented before its emergency Federal scheduling in 1984. The growing holistic health movement in the West has brought on a slew of new, FDA-sanctioned research in the US and Europe on the health and mind expansion benefits of psychedelic substances including psilocybin, LSD, MDMA, DMT (Dimethyltryptamine) and cannabis. Given our experiential inclination toward spirituality, it makes sense that we would seek to expand our consciousness and enhance our relationships through the use of psychedelic substances. In spite of ongoing sanctioned research, all of these substances are still federally illegal at the highest level in the US (Schedule I), making it hard to accurately portray what percentage of people are using psychedelics to augment their sexual connections and experiences – but we know it is happening to some degree.

We also know from a handful of multiple studies co-sponsored by MAPS (the Multidisciplinary Association of Psychedelic Studies) and other educational institutions across the globe that MDMA-assisted psychotherapy is extremely effective for reducing PTSD for trauma survivors (at an unprecedented rate of 83 per cent!) including sexual trauma survivors. A 2017 study published in the *Journal of Psychopharmacology* showed that MDMA can also enhance people's communication abilities, and ongoing studies are examining its effectiveness in couples' therapy.[83] In 2016, Katie Anderson from the Psychology Department at London South Bank University coined the term "MDMA Bubble" to refer to the "protective casing" that a couple develops when the medicine takes hold and they can begin to talk safely about the issues in their relationship.[84] While Anderson referred to patients who take the medicine in an office under the supervision of a therapist, the use of MDMA to enhance closeness and relational safety has been well documented, at least anecdotally.[85] Dee Dee Goldpaugh, a psychotherapist who specializes in sex positive psychotherapy with LGBTQ and polyamorous individuals, gave a sold-out talk on psychedelic sex therapy at the New York *Sexuality Speaker Series* in 2016. She explained why MDMA has so much potential for the couples' therapy of the near future:

It is highly effective in reducing and eliminating PTSD symptoms with very limited duration of treatment for clients who are survivors of assault or childhood sexual abuse. It induces extremely pleasurable sensation in the body allowing clients to feel being fully "embodied." It increases empathy and reduces shame, facilitating clients to experience their body as a safe place to be. In couples' work, we have evidence to suggest that MDMA can assist couples in communicating with each other in an unguarded way and to hear and hold their partner in a manner impossible to them when coming from a place of fear or defensiveness.[86]

Goldpaugh also argues that psilocybin's ability to reduce anxiety and increase openness to mystical and spiritual experiences could help assist with body image problems, sexual shame and sexual performance related issues. Furthermore, she predicts that in the future, psychedelics might even be used to treat sex offenders, citing a 2015 report on Brazilian prisoners finding lasting attitude change and developing remorse for their crimes after consuming ayahuasca tea while in prison.[87] We may see many psychologists administering psychedelic sex therapy in the next few years, and I predict it will become quite popular.

Is Sex a Spiritual Experience? Notes from the Ancient Wisdom Traditions

The notion of sex as a spiritual experience is certainly nothing new. Even our modern gurus and new age spiritualists have pulled from ancient understandings to explain the spiritual and energetic powers of sexuality. For example, in *Sex Matters: From Sex to Superconsciousness* (1978), Osho (real name Chandra Mohan Jain) explains:

> [U]ntil the naturalness of sex is accepted wholeheartedly, nobody can love anybody. I want to say to you that sex is godly. The energy of sex is divine energy, godly energy. That is why this energy creates a new life. It is the greatest, most mysterious force of all. Drop this antagonism toward sex. If you ever want love to shower you in your life, renounce this conflict with sex. Accept sex blissfully. Acknowledge its sacredness.[88]

Author Anaiya Sophia explains in *Sacred Sexual Union* (2013) how the concept of a sacred energetic union of two "soul halves" has been featured across Christianity, Tibetan Buddhism, Kabballah and tantra in Hinduism, and that it reflects "a way to progress in love toward God" (we will talk more about these soul halves in chapter 7).[89] Likewise, in *Jewel in the Lotus* (1987), authors Sunyata Saraswati and Bodhi Avinasha detail how tantric yoga uses "the most powerful energy we know – sexual energy – to penetrate the spiritual realms". They further explain that "the tantric masters discovered that prolonged sexual union produces super-sensitivity to the energies in and around the lovers."[90]

So where are these thinkers getting these ideas about spiritual sex? Well, from the past of course! When we look back across ancient human history, we discover a legacy of empowerment, knowledge and deep wisdom about the energetic forces of sex residing deep within our collective unconscious. While many of these techniques had been nearly forgotten, as our society continues to evolve toward sex positive attitudes, and as we become increasingly likely to search for spiritual meaning in these mundane areas of life, we are seeing a resurgence in many of these formerly sacred beliefs and practices.

For example, prior to the advent of Christianity, cultures like ancient Rome, Greece and Egypt had glorified sexuality as an empowering, important part of daily lives. Preserved ancient ruins like the city of Pompeii (complete with penis carvings in the street and hundreds of brothels) highlight the fact that early sexuality was not hidden or shameful (even though it still exemplifies a patriarchal society where men retained power and control over women). And yet the controlling and restrictive view of sexuality imposed around the advent of Christianity persisted through the Crusades all the way up until the end of the Victorian era, and still exists in some of the more evangelical sects even today. But some followers of the Gnostic tradition believe Jesus Christ did not intend this level of sexual rigidity in his teachings, and some like Sophia (2013) even argue he was married to Mary Magdalene in a sacred union. Who knows, but if we turn back the clock to pre-Christianity, we glimpse an even more intriguing picture of spirituality, sex and health.[91]

The Tao of Love and Sex

In Asia, the tradition of Taoism has been passed down through written tradition for over 2,000 years, and oral traditions could actually be much older. Paramount to Taoism is the notion of sexuality as medicine, and the idea that harmony can be achieved through balancing masculine and feminine energies. This is done by working with "*Qi*", or life force energies. The Taoist symbol of the "yin/yang" reflects the balance of feminine and masculine elements, with harmony occurring between these elements internally, as well as through both partners being completely satisfied. Taoism is one of the first sexual wisdom traditions to emphasize the concept of "sex as medicine", highlighting a close link between longevity, health and lovemaking. Chang's (1977) *The Tao of Love and Sex* accentuates the three key principles of the Tao, which still seem almost revolutionary even by today's standards: The regulation of ejaculation, the understanding that male orgasm and ejaculation are not necessarily one and the same thing, and the importance of female satisfaction.[92]

Yes, you heard that right. For thousands of years, certain cultures have conceptualized sex as a spiritual healing practice. By controlling the flow of life force energies, followers of the Tao could enhance their sexual prowess and wellbeing. The first principle, the regulation of ejaculation, is a far cry from how many people envision it today. The practice of the Tao warned against forced ejaculation, or the idea that a man should ejaculate every time he has sex. They also explained how orgasm and ejaculation were not the same thing. By holding in his sperm, the man literally conserves his sexual Qi. It is therefore up to every man practising the Tao to find the right ejaculatory frequency to suit his age and physical condition. Even a younger man should only ejaculate two or three times in every ten lovemaking sessions according to the Tao (what do you think about that, guys?!), and as he gets older, that number should decrease even more. By retaining his ejaculate, a man can harness his sexual energy to ensure long-lasting lovemaking where his female partner can receive extensive pleasure every single time. Such mutual pleasure was thought to help balance the yin/yang energies of the individual and maximize his wellbeing. The Tao includes a variety of tips for prolonging male erection and orgasm without ejaculation, and many of these have been paralleled by modern sexologists, including the William Masters and Virginia Johnson "squeeze technique".[93]

The White Tigresses

Speaking of female satisfaction, for the ultra-secretive White Tigresses sect of Taiwan, sexual expression was treated as a catalyst for spiritual transformation and youthfulness. They teach that "sexual energy is why a person is born, and lack of it is why a person dies." Thanks to the groundbreaking insider report by Hsi Lai (a pseudonym) featured in *The Sexual Teachings of the White Tigresses* (2001), people in the West were offered a first-time look into this ancient wisdom tradition that teaches women how to maximize the health benefits of sexual energy.[94] Using almost exclusively oral sex techniques only (not intercourse), the White Tigresses see absorbing or consuming male sexual Qi (by ingesting their semen) as a pathway to youthfulness, vitality, longevity and even immortality. Their philosophy reaches the heart of a woman's sexuality and spirituality, explaining how "sex is like a drug: abusing it withers and destroys you, while using it correctly restores and preserves you."[95] They believe that giving oral sex is their spiritual portal to reversing the aging process, because through taking the man's penis and ejaculate into her mouth, a woman has symbolic control and power over that man and his energies.

The White Tigresses would often spend many years (and even lifetimes!) studying how to harness sexuality for their own longevity, putting the scope of the specific White Tigress sexual practices way beyond this chapter. If you love the idea, I encourage you to read the book. One of the elements that I find fascinating is how men of the Tao try to conserve their ejaculate, whereas the females of the White Tigress attempt to coax it out. So, does sperm have "healing" qualities, not only energetically but scientifically? Well, it depends upon who you ask. For example, Hsi Lai refers to an older study from the Hebrew University showing that semen applied to a woman's face and chest had a number of wellness benefits including reducing wrinkles and healing acne.[96] However, the results were not consistent for men. Newer research has shown that when ingested into the body, male semen can have antidepressant effects for women by enhancing the uptake of oxytocin (more on oxytocin in the next chapter).[97] And who could forget actress Cate Blanchett attributing her flawless skin to facials that contain EGF (epidermal growth factor) serum derived from Korean baby foreskins? Maybe the White Tigresses were on to something after all?

Neotantra

Most of us are familiar with a Western version of "tantric sex" aka *neotantra*, thanks mostly to celebrities like Sting or Russell Brand, as well as a host of sex gurus, television shows and magazine articles on the topic. Of course, this version of tantric sex, where couples move slowly while making love, increasing arousal and leading to very long, multiple orgasms, does have some roots in the ancient tantra, although it has definitely been modified for Western consumption, so to speak. Tantra itself is a discipline that stems back thousands of years in India designed to harness spiritual sex to expand consciousness and join together the masculine and feminine energies. The gender of the partners involved is irrelevant here: We can pursue the balance of masculine (giving) and feminine (receiving) energies within ourselves, as well as in our relationships. It is based upon the guiding principle that the greatest source of energy in the universe is sexual energy. Tantra itself comprises part of the greater spiritual practice of kriya yoga, based upon the ancient Hindu texts, that incorporates yogic meditation, mantra, mandalas, gurus, initiation and ritual worship.

Neotantra remains a popular trend in the West, thanks in part to the uptake in activities like kundalini yoga (a school of yoga influenced by the Shakti, or Goddess energy, and the tantra schools of Hinduism) and Pranayama (the formal practice of controlling the breath, which is the source of our vital life force). According to *Jewel in the Lotus*, there are several energetic byproducts of practising tantric sex, including rejuvenation of the body-mind-spirit connection, clairvoyance, deepening your relationship, psychotherapy, dream learning, and reprogramming your subconscious.[98] (If you're thinking "Great, I need to learn this!" Go for it! There are some resources listed in the recommended reading for you). Generally, neotantric practice focuses on slowly building intimacy and sexual energy: Ritual cleansing, meditation, yoga, staring deeply into your lover's eyes, practising tantric massage and slow, deliberate sensual touch all constitute parts of the process. People practising neotantra are often encouraged to explore sexual taboos, either through the switching of traditional gender norms (such as, the female takes the lead while the male is submissive) or through exploring kink like BDSM (Bondage/Discipline/Sadism/Masochism).

The Sexual Teachings of Quodoushka

The teachings of Quodoushka, a spiritual wisdom tradition which has been handed down by the Twisted Hair Elders of the Nagual Traditions, exemplify how Native American wisdom traditions have traditionally embraced sexuality. For thousands of years, they have taught a shamanic approach to sexuality that emphasizes healing sexual guilt and repression through illumination and knowledge. According to Quodoushka, "the Great Spirit gives us two gifts: One is free will, and the other is orgasm." Highlighted in Amara Charles's wonderful *The Sexual Practices of Quodoushka* (2011), there is a wealth of wisdom in these teachings about the many types of male and female genital anatomy (nine types for each) and how the structure of your genitals dictates the types of pleasure that you prefer to receive.[99]

Quodoushka entails detailed sexual healing practices that address removing energetic blockages and aligning the flow of sexual energy throughout the body. Charles explains how "for thousands of years, naguals and sages in various ancient cultures have known that sexual energy can heal imbalances and extend life."[100] In her book, Charles details at length the sexual healing processes involving the chakras (wheel in Hindu, defined as the spinning energy funnels of our etheric bodies), also known as chulas in Quodoshka, or turning wheels. While this can only serve as a jumping-off point, the idea is that our auric or etheric bodies are made up of points where energy either pools and radiates or remains clogged up and closed off. No matter where on the body these points are, the Quodoushka believe we can use sexual healing practices to open up the blockages so that energy can flow more freely. As someone who has the chakras tattooed on her arm (yes, really!) and who has written a little bit in the past about the role of the chakras in sexual healing, I find this a completely fascinating topic. I encourage you to read up on the Quodoushka approach yourself to see if it resonates for you.

Sexual Consciousness: Where Sex and Energy Meet

If this brief review of ancient sexual wisdom traditions has taught you one thing, it should be how cultures across the globe have naturally sought to harness sexual energy for the purposes of healing, wellness and longevity.

But is this something most of us actually want? Judging by our spiritual inclinations toward health and wellness, it seems very likely. Our desire for more expansive knowledge and healing also explains the exponential rise in the popularity of these techniques. We talked at the start of the chapter about finding meaning as the old world comes crashing down around us, but how does spiritual sex fit into that picture of what is new and what is to come?

I believe that as we redefine sex and love, each of us travels a unique journey to develop our own sense of *Sexual Consciousness*. What does that mean? Think about it like this: Consciousness is defined as *the state or quality of awareness, or, of being aware of something within oneself*. Thus, "sexual consciousness" refers to developing a complete awareness of ourselves as sexual beings, not only in the physical sense, but also through the depths of the creative, alchemical and transformative energy we truly possess. It refers to our intuitive awareness and introspection into the ever-changing meanings of sex and intimacy in our lives. And remember, we are not talking about religion – or even about "spirit", really. We're talking about *energy*. Sexual consciousness itself also has nothing to do with dogma or beliefs. It is not contained within any one culture, ethnic group, nation state, gender or society. Sexual consciousness is something that all humans have possessed since the dawn of time. While we may have forgotten what the ancients once knew about sexual consciousness, we are starting to remember as we begin to redefine our attitudes to love.

Sexual consciousness must include our awareness of our intimate partners. We might ask, how is this person's energy affecting me? Case in point: This quote by Lisa Chase Patterson has been widely circulating over the past few years describing how when we have sex, we are not only merging bodies but also merging energies or auric fields:

> Pay attention to whom you share your intimate energy with. Intimacy at this level intertwines your aural energy with the aural energy of the other person. These powerful connections, regardless of how insignificant you think they are, leave spiritual debris; particularly within people who do not practice any type of cleansing. Physical, emotional or otherwise … I always say, never sleep with someone you wouldn't want to be.[101]

This passage is usually followed by instructions for clearing the aura, including Epsom salt baths, smudging (with sage), swimming in water, spending time in sunlight, as well as auric meditation, auric healing and aura readings. From this line of thinking, if you have sex with one person, and that person has had sex with ten people this year, then energetically, you may be absorbing the debris of all 11 partners into your energetic space or auric field. Much like the spread of STIs (sexually transmitted infections) then, so too can we potentially pick energetically or spiritually transmitted ailments if we are sleeping with the wrong people.

Now, this might be true. And you might have even experienced it! There is absolutely no way at present to prove or disprove the notion of energetic sexual contagions because much of our empirical data collection and analytical tools would have a challenging time measuring this phenomenon. But it would follow that as we elevate our sexual consciousness, we become more selective about who we choose to share and merge our energies with. We might decide not to have sex with someone who is extremely physically attractive because we can also discern that they may be emotionally/mentally/ energetically unattractive. However, we can only learn about these boundaries by making mistakes. How can we know how it feels to have sex with someone who is energetically unhealthy for us unless we first experience and know what it feels like? I'm fairly certain that most of the people reading this book have probably slept with someone who ended up not being such a great person or a great match for them … Does that mean our energy is permanently damaged? Of course not!

As we assess our potential partners, becoming sexually conscious beings means we must each build an honest, open awareness of ourselves. We need to stop lying to ourselves when we know better about what we want! So, what if you wanted to hook up with someone who does not have the best energy for you? Own it! To hell with plausible deniability, just stay accountable for the choices that you make and integrate them into your current identity so that you can keep growing. If we continue avoiding our true sexual desires, identities and feelings, then energetic meaningful sex will continue to elude us. Think about what you really want sexually. Do you know you want to go deep with someone and begin to unlock the healing power of sex? Do you want to get all tantric about it? Maybe you just want to start off by going deep with yourself? Or do you just want to keep it breezy and have some fun? Clear intentions lead to right action, so as long as you take the time for introspection and connecting with your truth, your journey to sexually conscious super bomb sex has already begun. Congrats!

And while we know that orgasm isn't the entire goal of spiritual sex, we also know that it's fundamentally important to our sexual satisfaction and wellbeing. Since our generation is already redefining everything about love, sex and relationships, we might as well as start rewriting the script about orgasms, too!

CHAPTER 5

REDEFINING ORGASM

Ancient healing traditions have taught for centuries that sexual activities can offer us life-giving, health-affirming benefits. Scientific research on orgasm heavily backs up this claim, with benefits ranging from physiological wellness, to reduced stress, to higher self-esteem and even to boosting intelligence. Whether you are having intercourse with a partner, experimenting with a friend, self-stimulating, masturbating to porn, fantasizing or playing with a sex toy or sex doll ... your orgasm is yours and there should never be any shame in having one! The ways we are experiencing orgasm is changing, creating a new story about how we like to do it, who we like to do it with and how it makes us feel. Indeed, the new frontiers of orgasm reflect the intersection of culture and technology with our progressive attitudes and our desires to orgasm. Thanks to new groundbreaking research on orgasm in the female brain, a wider acceptance of the many different types of orgasm, and a deeper understanding of why some people have not been able to orgasm, we are being presented with a glimpse of just how far conceptions of this universal human experience have shifted in our time.

Orgasm and Health: Yes, Yes, YES

Myriad scientific studies over the past few decades have proven that orgasms are very good for our health. In her groundbreaking book on the female orgasm, *Come As You Are* (2015), sex therapist Dr Emily Nagoski explains that orgasm is not just a physical, genital response but a "sudden involuntary release of sexual tension" that begins in the brain.[102] An orgasm itself can be difficult to describe, because it depends so much upon the individual and the context. Orgasmic experiences range from invoking a little sensation to feeling completely life altering. Maybe you've experienced both sides of the spectrum? We'll talk more about the range in human orgasm a little bit later in this chapter. But first, consider what we actually know about how truly positive it is for human beings to orgasm. With or without a partner, it appears that we still reap the health benefits!

Physiologically, the release of pleasure chemicals during orgasm has a variety of positive effects on the body. The excretion of oxytocin in the brain results in better sleep through its ability to regulate cortisol. A survey of 400 UK physicians on the topic of getting better sleep recently came to the conclusion, "Want a good night's sleep? Have more sex!"[103] Oxytocin also reduces anxiety and increases feelings of connectedness, which offers a biochemical basis for that "warm fuzzy feeling" we get right after sex.[104] Orgasms are also thought to elevate levels of DHEA, which reduce the effects of aging and can even help to regulate the immune system. When we orgasm, our blood vessels dilate, pumping more oxygen through the body, leading to that after-sex rosy "flush" that many people experience. The increase of oestrogen in the female body after orgasm also helps to boost our collagen levels, which offers a variety of skin and organ-restoring benefits.

Having sex raises our heart rate to a level comparable to working out, but no, sex does not give us the same benefits as running five miles in the gym. However, the heart rate nearly doubles during climax, meaning that we do receive some cardiovascular benefits when we orgasm. Indeed, studies have shown that regular orgasms reduce the risk of heart disease in men by as much as 36 per cent, although about 1 per cent of acute heart attacks are linked to sexual activity (usually in people with pre-existing heart conditions). One study published in the 2010 *American Journal of Cardiology* showed that men who had sex twice per week were less likely to develop heart disease than men who had sex less than once per month.[105] The dilation of blood vessels that occurs during orgasm also benefits heart health and can even lower blood pressure. Frequent ejaculation has also been correlated with a reduced rate of prostate cancer in men. Specifically, 21 ejaculations per month compared with 7 or fewer per month reduces a man's risk of prostate cancer.[106] (I wonder what the Taoists would have to say about that?!)

The physical benefits don't end here. One of the greatest effects of orgasm in both men and women is the profound potential for physical pain relief. In fact, orgasm actually increases a woman's pain threshold, suppressing pain without affecting sensitivity to touch (or as Komisaruk, Beyer-Flores and Whipple call it in *The Science of Orgasm*, "analgesia without anaesthesia").[107] Not only can orgasm help to relieve period cramps and pain in women, but a 2013 study showed that orgasm can actually help relieve some severe migraines and cluster headaches.[108]

The biochemical release of pleasure hormones like oxytocin during orgasm also does wonders for mental health. Orgasms are significant stress reduction tools: In one survey of over 2,000 women, nearly 40 per cent reported that they masturbated to help themselves relax.[109] Ever heard of cortisol, that pesky little stress hormone? Well the secretion of oxytocin after orgasm helps to bring down our cortisol levels, literally reducing our anxiety and making us feel less stressed out. Orgasms can also enhance our self-esteem, probably through the same process as relieving our stress. When we feel calm and relaxed, we feel better about ourselves and our lives.

Orgasms may even make us more intelligent by stimulating the growth of brain cells. Researchers found that prolonged sexual activity in lab rats led to enhanced cognitive function, including hippocampal abilities and promoting neurogenesis (aka, the growth of new brain cells).[110]

Whether these effects can be extrapolated to humans remains to be seen, but the research is certainly promising.

How We Are Redefining Orgasm

In light of our exposure to all of this new research on the benefits of orgasm, can we assume that we are having more sex than any generation before us? Not exactly. We might be having more orgasms, but not necessarily more sex with actual partners. Psychologist Jean Twenge made waves with her data analysis showing that millennials are actually having less sex than the older generations (like our parents) did when they were our age![111] While it is true that millennials are having more sex than any other generation currently alive on the planet (about 80 times per year on average, compared with 20 times per year of people over 60), we are having less intercourse than previous generations did at our age (we're having intercourse about nine fewer times per year than adults in 1989, to be exact).

What is going on here? How can we explain the lack of sexual frequency in a generation that has had more access to sexual materials and embodies more sexually permissive attitudes than any before them? The way I see it, we might not be having quite as much intercourse, but we are having different types of sex, including oral sex, anal sex and self-stimulation. We are changing what it means to orgasm, and with whom and how frequently. For example, the same analysis showing millennials had less sex also showed that compared with past generations, millennials have a greater number of sexual partners, were more permissive of non-marital sex and were more likely to have had sex with an acquaintance.[112] We are also much more likely than past generations to masturbate, to experiment with sex, and to integrate technology into the bedroom. Thanks to the vast array of available pornography, sex toys and virtual sex options like sexting, webcamming and virtual partners, we don't really need a partner on deck to make us orgasm. We've actually become excellent at doing it ourselves! This is empowering in a lot of ways, as long as we don't end up on that slippery slope discussed in chapter 3 of never needing to have any intimate interactions with other humans ever again. But more on that in a moment.

Is it any surprise that we love sexting and self-pleasuring? In 2017, the SKYN condom company conducted a massive survey of millennials in the US and found that half had sent or received a nude 'sext' at least once per week.[113] Living in an increasingly fragmented and busy world where we don't always have opportunities to meet up (or maybe because so many of us are forced to still live with our parents), we rely upon technology to turn us on and excite us when we don't have our partners in front of us. Eighty-nine per cent of women in the survey also said they could orgasm through masturbation and did so on a regular basis, which is much higher than the sex studies of the past would have you believe. According to a TENGA survey of 1,200 American adults, millennials are masturbating much more frequently than other generations, about 15 times per month compared with 12 times per month for Gen-X-ers and 7 times per month for baby boomers.[114] The stigma of masturbation being a "bad" thing has definitely fallen by the wayside in our generation, as we were by far the most comfortable generation in the survey to talk about masturbation. One in five of the millennials in the survey even said they masturbate with the intention of getting better at sex!

Now I know what you're thinking: Good sex should require some level of commitment, intimacy and vulnerability with another human, and here we go again finding another selfish way to circumvent all of this! To that I say, hold your horses. While it's true that we masturbate more than anyone in modern history, we have to consider our sexuality in the context of our lives and environments. We have grown up with technology that offers us unlimited options of sexual partners, fuck buddies and masturbation materials. This means that many of us have limited attention spans when it comes to committing to a long-term relationship, because we can't help but scroll and scan for the bigger, better deal (technology and social media have literally taught us do this, as we'll discuss more about later in the book). Many of us also still live at home with our parents (talk about a sexual buzz kill, unless the prospect of getting caught turns you on, of course), we work multiple jobs often at strange hours and we are inherently distrustful of sexual connections because we have seen in light of the #MeToo movement how sex can become coercive, stressful or harmful to our wellbeing. By self-pleasuring, we are reducing our sexual risk factor for STIs and unwanted pregnancy. Are we really to blame as the harbingers of the doom of sex? I've even stumbled upon the headlines, "Millennials Are Ruining America's Sex Life", "Millennials Are Killing Sex" and "Millennial Sex Sucks".[115] But is there another side that the haters haven't considered?

We might be having less vaginal intercourse than previous generations, but I doubt we are having fewer orgasms. We are having different kinds of sex and orgasms: For example, the SKYN Lifestyles survey showed that we are much more likely than older generations to have multiple orgasms, with nearly half of males and females reported having two or more orgasms during a single sexual encounter. We are also way more likely to have experimental sex, like anal sex. Nearly 1 in 4 millennial females had received anal sex and 1 in 6 millennial males had received anal sex, much higher than the national average.[116] And yes, before you ask, a woman can orgasm from penetrative anal sex, with some women reporting intense pleasure from how the penis hits the G spot from behind. For example, I have a girlfriend who can only orgasm from the combination of clitoral stimulation with anal penetration. And many men can experience intense prostate orgasms from receiving anal sex – even without having an erection, which may explain why pegging (female to male receptive anal sex) has been trending so hard lately. I would have never known when I bought my first strap-on a decade ago that today, it would become a mainstream sex toy sold extensively on Amazon.

Speaking of Amazon, a 2018 survey showed that over half of millennials would rather "give up sex" than give up their Amazon

Prime memberships.[117] But take that with a pinch of salt. We have to wonder if we would "give up sex" because we orgasm so well alone, rather than assuming we just have bad sex or hate sex. After all, the survey didn't ask about giving up masturbation. Maybe Amazon streaming services offer us something that we can't do ourselves, whereas we know that we can get an orgasm just fine? For our generation, less sex might actually equal more orgasms. But are all orgasms created equally?

Are All Orgasms Created Equally?

One of the funny things about orgasms is how they represent so much more than just a one-size-fits-all approach, especially for women. In *Come As You Are*, Nagoski details a variety of orgasms that women have described to her, including:

- Orgasm from clitoral stimulation.
- Orgasm from anal stimulation.
- Orgasm just from breast stimulation.
- Orgasm from having her toes sucked.
- Orgasm where her partner slowly and gently stroked fingertips upward along her outer labia.
- Orgasm without any genital stimulation when she was giving her partner oral sex.[118]

The crucial message here is that one type of orgasm is not better or more "normal" than another. According to Nagoski, female sexual desire and arousal has traditionally been regarded as "male sexual arousal lite", meaning that we have used the same metrics to measure men's sexuality as women's.[119] We assume that heterosexual vaginal intercourse is the most important sex, because that is what "gets men off" (and what makes babies!). But what really matters, at least according to Nagoski, is the release of sexual tension that happens regardless of the type of sex that leads to the release. The parts of the body that were stimulated are less important than the overall feeling of what happened, and the individual's understanding of it. Sometimes we orgasm in our sleep. Sometimes we orgasm riding a horse or bicycle. Sometimes women orgasm during childbirth. There are even scientific accounts of atypical orgasms that happen during epileptic seizures or as the result of stimulating the spine during chronic pain therapy, or from neurochemical stimulation applied directly to the brain.[120] Just because our brain tells us that we had an orgasm does not mean we were necessarily turned on or had a profound sexual experience. Sometimes we feel pleasure and release with our orgasms, and sometimes we don't. We will talk more a little bit later about why this is the case.

Suffice it to say that there are lots of different types of orgasms, and most of them depend upon the context and emotional/psychological landscape of the individual at any given moment. If you are having sex but unable to focus because you are busy thinking about that job interview in the morning, it might be hard to experience a completely ecstatic release, which is usually the only one we picture when we think about orgasm: The complete body shuddering glorious joyful release of all of that energy. We don't always have that. But when we do, explains Nagoski, it usually happens out of a sense of *integration*, of every part of us working together to surrender and lose ourselves in that moment of complete release.[121]

Energetically speaking, are there different types of orgasms? According to the Quodoushka tradition, some orgasms have the power to energize us, while others drain our energy and leave us feeling depleted. How can we tell the difference? Our attitudes and approaches to sex can predict the healing benefits of our orgasms, and whether we will feel energized or depleted after sex. When we are distracted, overthinking, blaming others for our unhappiness, always complaining about wanting more, putting our demands and expectations on others, having obsessive sexual thoughts, feeling resentment toward our partner(s), or staying in an unhappy, unsatisfying relationship, then sex and orgasms can actually drain us. Charles explains that these draining sexual experiences are different from having "high level orgasms" which can "take us into expanded states of consciousness where our hearts open and love flows unconditionally. We gain a direct connection to Source and feel oneness with everything."[122]

How do we access these expanded states of consciousness through orgasm? Charles asserts that our physical health and overall lifestyle are predictors of high-level orgasms. From this perspective, our orgasms become energetically beneficial when we are living a balanced life, including following a healthy diet, exercising regularly and keeping a playful, open attitude where we remain present with everyone we encounter. Charles recommends that we must slow down, destress and observe all openings for intimacy. Specifically, by maintaining what she calls "a neutral *Witness-Observer* perspective" (where we observe the energy of our lovemaking without attachment or expecting a certain outcome), we "savour what is happening more than what we project or pretend is going to happen".[123] Of course, this can be challenging when we have had another lie shoved down our throats: That all good sex must end in orgasm.

In spite of our rising awareness of the importance of the female orgasm, around 5 to 15 per cent of women have never had an orgasm, making it the second reason why women seek treatment for sexual problems behind sexual desire itself.[124] Is there anything wrong with a woman who has never had an orgasm? No!

Rejecting the Expectation of "Achieving" Orgasm

As we discussed at the start of the book, so much of what we think we know about sex is fake old news we've been taught by a crumbling patriarchal system that no longer serves us. This could not be more relevant than when it comes to the conception of orgasm as the be-all, end-all purpose of sex. How many times has someone felt like a failure because their partner wasn't able to orgasm? How many times has it sparked fights, insecurities and conflicts in your life, or led to the end of a relationship altogether? Our insane focus on work ethic and productivity has programmed us to believe that we must accomplish goals at all times, especially when it comes to sex. If our partner didn't orgasm, then did we fail to please them or to do our "job"? Absolutely not. Sex and orgasms are not about a job, they are supposed to be an enjoyable intimate experience. As we begin to embrace more sex positive attitudes, we realize that sexual interactions themselves have never been just about orgasm: They are all about *pleasure*!

We are entering a time in our collective sexual development where it becomes crucial to reframe orgasm in terms of our intentions to give pleasure as opposed to performing on command and delivering orgasms on cue. Especially for women, it is simply not going to happen every single time in the context of intercourse. Most women have a hard time orgasming from vaginal sex alone, and some cannot orgasm at all. Can you still enjoy sex even if you are not orgasming? Of course! The pleasure that comes from stimulating physical touch and connection with our partners is sometimes even better than the orgasm itself. According to Quodoushka teachings, "paradoxically, the way to enjoy consistently higher levels of orgasm is to let go of trying to get them."[125] Ironically then, the more we stop aiming for this goal, the more easily we can achieve it. We can no longer allow the pressure to deliver orgasms to squeeze the joy out of sex! We all deserve better!

For years in our culture (and even in the study sexology itself), it has been assumed that vaginal intercourse was somehow the "pinnacle" and goal of all types of lovemaking. Yes, this idea stems from a model which wrongly assumes that what pleasures the male from an evolutionary perspective should therefore also inherently pleasure the female. However, most women do not actually orgasm during vaginal intercourse. This explains why as many as 9 in 10 women who masturbate do so without any vaginal penetration, usually focusing exclusively on clitoral stimulation.[126] Women, if we're great at masturbating but rarely do so using the vagina, are we really surprised at the fact that vaginal sex alone doesn't always make us orgasm? This discussion is in no way intended to shame or discount the women who do orgasm from vaginal sex. It is more about reframing our expectations so that we never again feel broken or bad if vaginal sex doesn't make us orgasm, just like we shouldn't shame men for being "minute men" (as Missy Elliott put it) and coming too quickly.[127]

Orgasm and the Female Brain

One of the most pressing issues that has emerged in the field of sexology is why women seem to struggle more than men when it comes to orgasm. Yes, we can blame the patriarchy and the fake old news of the Victorian age for creating an environment where women were not allowed to embrace themselves as sexual beings or enjoy their sexuality. But what if there is something more going on? What if men and women are physiologically different in the ways that we experience orgasm? And yet, because scientists for so long have assumed that the male model is "correct" and that female sexuality could be explained using this model, what could we have missed?

In *Come As You Are*, Nagoski puts forward the thesis of the "*dual control model*" of sexuality: Namely, that everyone's sexual arousal and response is dictated by the "*brakes*" and "*accelerators*" in our brains. She explains how people have a sexual "exciter" that responds to sexually relevant information, including anything we touch, hear, see, smell or taste that turns us on. Conversely, our sexual response is also dictated by the sexual "inhibitors" that respond to potential threats (which can be anything we see, hear, smell, touch, taste or imagine that gives us a good reason not to be turned on right now).[128]

You might be reading this and asking, what does this have to do with orgasm? Well, simply put, people's ability to orgasm requires an equation of more sexual exciters activated and with fewer brakes engaged. Because of the fake old news women are told about their sexuality, it can sometimes take a lot more of the sexual accelerators to turn us on. While Nagoski explains that this is an individual difference and there isn't a lot we can do to change our inherent sexual accelerators or brakes, it does help to explain why some women don't orgasm every time, if at all. She posits, if we raised 100 girls in a sex positive culture that teaches them to embrace and trust their sexual bodies, would we see more women pulling their feet off the brakes and slamming them onto the accelerators? Maybe. But:

> Even in a sex positive culture, women with more sensitive brakes and less sensitive accelerators would need extra sexy stimulation before arousal sparked into desire.[129]

In other words, we can't blame culture for everything, just like we can't blame physiology for everything. As discussed earlier, we are always working with and trying to overcome the interaction between nature and nurture. But how does the brain play into this?

Differences in Female and Male Arousal and Response

As it turns out, people experience a disparity in how turned on their physical body is versus how turned on their brains say they are. Research shows that men have about a 50 per cent overlap in what their genitals respond to as "sexually relevant" and what their brains respond to as "sexually appealing". About half of the time, a man will get a hard-on in response to stimulation that his brain finds sexually arousing. The other half? His penis literally has a mind of its own. But women only have about a 10 per cent overlap between how their genitals respond to sexually relevant information and what their brain tells them is sexually appealing!

This is why you might hear plenty of stories from women in your life (I know I have!) about feeling sexually turned on, but not being able to get wet down there, or about being wet for no reason and not feeling turned on at all. I've even heard stories about women who were raped or sexually assaulted and were either wet during the attack or even had an orgasm. Women's physical sexual response has *very little* to do with their neurological processing and how they feel emotionally! This is one of men's and women's greatest differences when it comes to understanding the science of orgasm: The relationship between the genitals and the central nervous system (the brain) is fundamentally different for men and women. If you are a woman reading this book, do you relate with this finding? If we know that in women, about 90 per cent of the time our bodies' sexual arousal and our mind's sexual desire do not match up, I believe that we can work with this knowledge to explain the sexual situations of our pasts, and connect more deeply with how we experience this disconnect in the present and future, starting with the new and exciting ways that we are getting ourselves off.

Vibrat-orGasms Galore

Nearly half of all adult women in America own vibrators, and most of us would claim that in terms of clitoral stimulation, they offer the easy accessibility for quick and enjoyable orgasms. There are so many vibrators and sex toys for women's orgasm out there now, it can be hard to keep track. From vibrating dildos to cute devices that literally suck on your clitoris, to the Magic Wand, to devices that don't even vibrate at all, there is truly something for everyone. One of the ways that that women are changing the nature of orgasm is through the alleged "closing" of the gender gap. Women are actually finding ways to orgasm more frequently during sex than ever before, thanks in part to new specially designed sex toys. A relatively new toy called the Dame which attaches hands free to the clitoris for use during penetrative heterosexual sex has gained widespread popularity, raising hundreds of thousands of dollars during only a few months on Kickstarter in 2016. The premise? This device enables women to level the playing field to come from clitoral orgasms during sex. While women currently reflect only about one-third of the global $15 billion per year sex toy industry, this number is expected to skyrocket as increasing numbers of women are designing toys for the sole purpose of closing the orgasm gap and enhancing women's pleasure.[130]

Some women fear that using a vibrator on their clitoris will erode their sensitivity, but there is no hard evidence to support this claim. Rather, due to the intense and rapid stimulation of vibrators, we do find that we can shorten how long it takes to orgasm. And then, when we find ourselves with physical partners, or when we are self-stimulating, we are reminded that it takes much longer to orgasm. I know plenty of women who have sworn themselves off vibrators and only masturbate using their fingers because they want it to be more reminiscent of the real thing. Is a vibrator orgasm any better or worse for you than a self-stimulated one or one with a partner? No. Should we feel shame that we need a tool to orgasm or that we want to use it with a partner? Of course not. We can all do whatever we want. And at least more and more people are starting to realize this by demanding a variety of toy options! No matter your gender or sexuality, you deserve pleasure in whatever way it comes most naturally, including masturbation, toys and other tools. Just by being an adult human, you owe it yourself to experience and unlock the pleasure of your body without shame or apology.

More than Pee? Female Ejaculation

Before we become male or female (or something different for intersexed people) in utero, all humans start out with the same organs. In science, we call these *homologous* organs. The glans or "head" of the penis and the clitoris both begin as the same organ, as does the male prostate and the glands that comprise the female G spot. This explains why some women can ejaculate, because men and women share the same homologous glands for it, even though they change during our development in utero.

One of the most frequent questions I am asked regarding women's orgasm is whether the liquid that is sometimes excreted from the female urethra during sex and/or orgasm is "just pee" or something else. Some women do in fact experience ejaculatory orgasms during which they "squirt" liquid similar to how men ejaculate. I'm happy to live in a sex positive world now where we can have an open dialogue about female ejaculation, even though it remains controversial both socially and scientifically. For example, Great Britain actually banned female ejaculation or "squirting" in porn in 2016 (with all the extreme weirdness in porn, I can only say, WTF?), because it resembles urine and all types of piss porn are banned in the UK at the time of writing.

However, some female ejaculate *is* more than "just pee", and according to the *Journal of Sexual Medicine* (2011), is excreted from a female's Skene's glands during orgasm, containing small amounts of PSA (prostate specific antigen).[131] PSA is also found in men's ejaculate and helps the sperm to swim. A 2014 French study looked at seven women who reported recurrent and massive fluid emissions during sex and found some interesting results.[132] Using ultrasound, the researchers showed that although the participants' bladders were completely empty before sex, they filled themselves up when the women were sexually excited and then emptied after the orgasmic ejaculation, proving that yes, the ejaculate contains pee – but the researchers also found traces of fluid picked up from the Skene's glands.

My sex positive self can't help but think, who cares even if it is 100 per cent urine, because clearly this is an important sexual experience and huge sexual release for those who have it (not to mention a turn-on for many others, regardless of gender). Some of these studies have been confounded by the fact that some women who ejaculate do not necessarily mark it as the same as orgasm – sometimes it is a completely different sensation altogether. With this whole hullaballoo over female ejaculation we just need to remind ourselves that people experience sexual pleasure differently and that is cool with us. But I do hope that science and research will continue to shed light on exactly what is happening physiologically and psychologically here. Speaking of innovation, do we have any clue what the orgasms of the future might look and feel like?

Will Mindgasms Become the Orgasms of the Future?

In the near future, technology promises to alter the very nature of sex as an orgasmic experience. Scientists and futurists predict that soon, sex will become a solely mental experience we could achieve through plugging electrodes into our brains or using advanced virtual reality or other sophisticated stimulatory technologies. Dawson and Owsianik (2016) propose that such "pleasure implants" will be connected to stimulate the pleasure centres of the brain, "bringing people to new orgasm heights and allowing them to experience the orgasms of one or several people at the same time".[133] Likewise, in his 2015 short film, *The Future of Sex*, futurist Jason Silva claims that "the future of sex is like the future of art: More immersion, more intensity, deeper subjectivity. Orgasms and mindgasms for all!"[134]

Now you're probably asking, what on earth is a *mindgasm* and how can I get one? Or several? Silva is alluding to the nature of our technology to bridge gaps between people and forge deeper mental connections. He predicts that in the near future, we will orgasm so much harder from simulated in-brain technology than from other people that we won't require the physical act of sex itself to satiate ourselves. Silva posits that our future offers the potential of virtual reality sex where we lose ourselves so completely in pleasure that rubbing our bodies against each other to orgasm will seem like a faint memory! Dawson and Owsianik agree, arguing that by 2027, brain-to-brain interfaces (like those featured in the 1994 film *Demolition Man*, or am I showing my age?) will allow partners to stimulate each other to reach orgasm directly, without any physical touch. Such a process would unfold via the use of neural headsets that record wavelengths that can produce "erotic mind melding" and even thought sharing.[135]

Scientifically, the idea of a mindgasm is certainly nothing new, as there have been a multitude of anecdotal reports and even books written about people with the ability to make themselves or others orgasm completely non-physically. Across tantra, hypnosis psychology and other varied esoteric traditions, attaining an orgasm without even touching your genitals has indeed been a story for the ages. In *The Science of Orgasm* (2006), Komisaruk reports that subjects who felt that they had achieved a mindgasm (not a stimulated orgasm) showed brain activity in the exact same regions of the brain during an fMRI (functional magnetic resonance imaging) as those who were stimulated to orgasm by physical genital contact.[136] Some of the women in his studies could actually "think" themselves to orgasm (aka "*thinking-off*"), a phenomenon which has been captured and milked by numerous media outlets, sex gurus, orgasm workshops and so on. In 2016, hypnotist Mark Cunningham claimed it was possible for women to think themselves to orgasm using the power of suggestion, a meditation process of deep rhythmic breathing and expanding and contracting the pelvic floor with Kegel exercises.[137]

If mindgasms are indeed already possible for some people, then it is hardly a stretch to assume that technology may soon be able to easily and effectively stimulate our brains to have orgasms every single time. Of course, this begs the question of whether it is innate or comfortable for humans to completely relinquish the desire for real-life physical contact, no matter how immersive electrodes in our brains may feel. Then again, if we were to grow up in a world where physical sex was an ancient taboo, maybe mindgasms would feel more enjoyable than stimulated physical ones? We already know that chemical brain stimulation as well as spinal stimulation has been shown to create unexpected, atypical orgasms in some people. From a public health perspective, this type of mental-only sexual connection means fewer physical partners, lessened exposure to STIs and health risks, and lowered incidence of pregnancy. Are you excited about a near future where sex occurs only in our minds, on some kind of ethereal plane that we can unlock as our technology continues to advance? And that it might even be qualitatively and quantitatively better than the real thing?

A Holistic Model for Enhancing Orgasm

This chapter would not be complete without a model or philosophy aimed at how to reach a state of integration between mind, body and spirit to enhance our experiences of orgasm. Eyal Matsliah's *Orgasm Unleashed* (2015) suggests a five-step holistic transformational model for unleashing your best orgasm:

> *Reflect:* Look at where you are now. Who are you? What are your limiting beliefs of your orgasmic experience?
> *Know:* What do you need to know about your body and the types of orgasm you can experience?
> *Embody:* What can you actually do to completely embody a greatest orgasmic release? What techniques can expand your experience?
> *Receive:* Do you feel it's ok to ask for and receive help? How can others assist in your healing and on your orgasmic journey?
> *Transform:* Your orgasmic practice can change your life. What lifestyle changes would support your sexuality?[138]

While asking yourself these questions won't necessarily lead to having more ecstatic orgasms, I appreciate this process because it reflects the inherent subjectivity in all of our sexual experiences: We already know that people don't orgasm in the same ways or even experience pleasure in the same ways, but if we want a complete orgasmic release it has less to do with our partners and more to do with our balanced relationships with ourselves. If we truly must integrate our mental and physical comfort, our psychological state and our general acceptance of ourselves in order to have a mind-blowing orgasm, then we can start by asking ourselves these questions right now. By really living in the moment, and rejecting the idea of expectations and outcomes, we can begin to cultivate an orgasmic mindset that can enable us to have deeply satisfying orgasms.

We've learned that we are redefining orgasm, just like we are changing everything else in our sexual worlds. But as individuals, how do we cope with all of these changes while still remaining mentally healthy and true to ourselves?

CHAPTER 6
LEARNING TO HEAL

Throughout this book so far, we have been exploring how our generation has systematically deconstructed and rewritten the script about love, sex and relationships. I believe that on some deeper, intuitive and/or metacognitive level, you already know who you are sexually, you know your values, and you know what you want out of life and relationships. As the world feels like it is shifting so rapidly around us, it is important to really work on ourselves so that we can remain present, heal our traumas and continue to evolve to become the sexual beings we were born to be. And crucially, if we want to fall in love and/or cultivate more sex positive relationships in our lives, we must do this work on ourselves first.

If this exploration into our sex positive attitudes has taught us anything, it should be that most of us want the same things: We want to be loved. We want to be heard. We want to be accepted. We want close connections, but only with people who respect our independence. We embrace variety and diversity. We want to experiment. But most of all, we want to *heal*.

If we really intend to replace the old narrative with something more sex positive and authentic to our real lives, then we have to be honest with ourselves about our hang-ups, our shortcomings and the traumas that we continue to carry, imparted upon us from spending most of our lives in a society that has been in relative upheaval. We can't close the book on that old story if we're still very much writing it. In order to become beacons of light who can spread our sex positive beliefs, there is healing, release and forgiveness that needs to happen for all of us. And guess what? I'm right there alongside you, trying to do the work.

Everyone – Every. Single. Person. Alive – has experienced some form of conscious or unconscious trauma about sex, love and/or relationships. Maybe the reason why you picked up this book to begin with was because the #MeToo movement triggered an awareness of your own sexual trauma and you are looking for healing. Or maybe you've just always felt like there was something "wrong" with your sexuality or ugly about your sexual body. Maybe you felt like you were born in the wrong body/as the wrong sex or gender. Maybe you felt ashamed to be gay or bisexual. Maybe your parents' relationship scarred you so badly that you're terrified of getting close to anyone. Maybe a relationship with a narcissist shredded your self-esteem. Maybe you've never had an orgasm. Maybe you got an STI or got pregnant as a teen and the shame has haunted you ever since. Maybe you identify as technosexual, polyamorous or pansexual and you always felt confused and alone. In the time of #MeToo, more and more people are coming forward and sharing their diverse stories, making this a time of healing now more than ever.

We all have something deep inside that is holding us back from feeling truly empowered, self-confident and at peace with who we are as sexual human beings. I can't possibly tell you exactly what it is for you, but you can. You already know. I shared my story in the introduction, from being slut shamed as a teen, to severe uterine problems that almost killed me and forced the removal of my uterus way before I was ready. But when it comes to you, I just want you to know that whatever happened to you doesn't define you. Whatever traumas you have experienced, remember this: You don't have to think of yourself as a victim. You are a survivor. A quote attributed to Carl Jung reminds us that, "I am not what happened to me; I am what I choose to become."

When it comes to healing sexual trauma, I could share with you various therapeutic approaches. And indeed, people have tried and had some success with everything from psychotherapy, to hypnosis, to somatic therapy, to energy work, to acupuncture to psychedelic medicine and beyond. I encourage you to pursue any and all avenues that resonate for you, now and forever. Yes, I could describe all of the options open to you (some of which are in the recommended reading) but what I'd really like to do is share with you some simple exercises that have worked for me, that you can begin doing right now. You don't have to pay a therapist or even leave your house. I can't promise that any of this will heal you, because only you can decide to turn yourself into the sexually empowered being that you already are deep inside. I only ask you to keep an open mind about starting the process of releasing the trauma.

Recognizing Programmed Self-Limiting Beliefs

Learned behaviour patterns offer fascinating insight into the human psyche. When we become conditioned by our families, institutions and our society, we internalize those beliefs and often act out models of them over and over again. When we find ourselves in relationship patterns (such as, always dating a bad boy, or always dating a woman who reminds you of your mother), we can become stuck in a rut where we are unable to grow as human beings. Many of us punish ourselves continuously without realizing we are doing it. We look at content online that makes us feel bad about ourselves. We compare ourselves to other people and feel worthless because we haven't achieved enough compared to everyone else. These are patterns of people who have been conditioned to have low self-esteem, often because of abuse that happens early in life. And just for the record, "abuse" doesn't always have to be physical abuse, it can manifest as a mental or psychological experience as well. (Find me someone with perfect parents who raised them without any issues and I'll write you a cheque for $1,000. It cannot be done.)

Imagine a man whose mother has Borderline Personality Disorder (BPD) which makes her emotionally confrontational and hostile. He might repeatedly date women who seem loving at first but as they become close, they may end up inflicting the same abuse and hostile energy upon him as his mother did. Why? It may actually feel comforting to seek out learned behaviour patterns even when they are harmful to us. Our brain associates the experience with a level of familiarity, and even though it makes us miserable inside, we keep doing it, over and over. Perhaps we subconsciously seek to repeat the same relationship patterns that were programmed into us as children.

Learned behaviour patterns often stem from *programmed self-limiting beliefs*, which are ideas that have been implanted into our subconscious minds through conditioning. Often, these beliefs are self-sabotaging and harmful to our growth and development. When it comes to love, and sex and relationships, some programmed self-limiting beliefs include:

- Nobody will ever love me.
- I should feel ashamed about my gender identity/sexual preferences/desires.
- Anyone who gets close to me will hurt me.
- I am not attractive.
- I deserve to be punished.
- My body is not a safe place.
- I can't let anyone see my true self.
- I deserve to be alone for the rest of my life.
- I can't trust anybody.

In *The Biology of Belief*, Dr Bruce Lipton makes an excellent argument that most of the subconscious programming of self-limiting beliefs happens before the age of seven. Subconsciously, we internalize the models that are presented to us as children, while our brains are still malleable. This is the same reason why when a child is exposed to a language before age seven, they will retain that language, but find it harder to retain if they started learning it as a teenager.[139]

To the extent that our minds retain these programmed self-limiting beliefs, Lipton argues that to reprogramme them we must first deconstruct them within the subconscious. He offers a number of different techniques for reprogramming subconcious patterning on his website (see link in recommended reading section).[140]

I believe that in addition to techniques to deprogramme our subconscious minds, we must also work within our conscious minds to recognize when we are engaging in a pattern that has been reinforced by self-limiting beliefs. We have to keep working through these patterns in order to notice them, and often, they might not be uncovered for decades. People can often perform huge amounts of mental gymnastics to protect themselves from really seeing these patterns, preferring to reside in the comfort that comes from being unwilling to change. But if you're reading this, then you probably are willing to change and actively seeking it out! If we really want to view these patterns with our conscious minds, we must engage in sort of willing dissociation where we can witness ourselves as both the observer and the object being observed (similar to the idea of the *witness-observer* presented by Quodoushka healing practices in the last chapter), so we become empowered and aware when we can see ourselves as both the participant of our behaviours and as the witness to them. Imagine your soul is watching your body and mind from a higher place where we can see the past, present and the future, based upon our current behaviours. Would you be able to recognize your learned behaviour patterns then? Of course you would. But how on earth can we achieve that level of self-observation for the sake of integration and healing?

In my experience, meditation and breathwork have been fundamental in observing myself from an outsider's perspective. When I drop into my meditative state, I am no longer justifying, lying to myself or playing mental gymnastics: I am observing all that is, without judgement of myself or anyone else. I become a passive observer to the movement of life all around me. This is a way that I can bring myself into a place of objectively observing my reality, as opposed to only believing the story I tell myself so that I do not have to grow, change or face the pain that I am carrying. There are so many different types of meditation out there: Transcendental, Vedic, Zen Buddhist and so on. And before you say, "I'm just not a meditator, I can't sit still that long I'll go crazy," please know that I said the same thing for years until I finally committed to trying it. You can start small, five minutes per day, and work your way up. I always recommend that new meditators start with breathwork first, before even trying visualization techniques. I strongly recommend Danny Penman's fabulous book *The Art of Breathing* as a great introduction.[141] Given that we are becoming increasingly distracted by technology and screens, we need meditation now more than ever to help us create a calm mind–body space for healing to take place.

Some people also like to use psychedelic medicine to reach the state of the witness-observer. While I can't recommend this without a physician's supervision because people's physiologies are so different, I have read anecdotal reports that for some people, the absolute breakthrough of a really intense acid trip, or an extreme k-hole dissociation, or 5 grams of mushrooms in a dark room (to paraphrase Terrence McKenna) offers a perspective of complete ego death. If meditation or psychedelic therapy just isn't your bag, consider "free writing" where you sit in front of the page and write whatever comes to mind in a stream of consciousness. This has to be with a pen and paper though, not in front of a screen or on a keyboard, because you are physically connecting your body to your energy and your flow. Just write whatever comes to mind, and usually this will impart whatever is clogging you up subconsciously. When you go back and read the stream later, you might start to pick out certain patterns in your thinking that you never considered before. Sometimes, the pattern or the programmed self-limiting beliefs will jump right off the page.

Acknowledging Trauma

Once we begin to recognize our programmed self-limiting beliefs, we need to address where they came from. Like the example of the mother with BPD in the last section, it is important to notice that some sort of trauma has taken place which has led to the programming of self-limiting beliefs in our brain, bringing out an inner critic with a hostile self-dialogue. And please note, even if the trauma happened after the age of seven, it can still lead to self-limiting beliefs and harsh inner critics. When we talk about sexual trauma, we often think of rape, incest and sexual abuse, but there are others forms of sexual trauma as well, like being kicked out of the house at 16 years old because you came out as gay, or being teased relentlessly in the locker room because of the size of your genitals or other parts of your sexual body. Or, you could have had such extreme problems with your sex organs that it almost ruined your life (ahem, this would be me).

It is not up to us to decide whose trauma was "worse". In reality, people rarely do this. On the contrary, most people who have experienced sexual trauma tend to minimize, deny or distance themselves from what happened. Therapists commonly hear phrases like, "it wasn't even that bad," or, "it was such a long time ago," or, "other people have had it so much worse I shouldn't even complain." Other times, people will blame themselves for what happened, internalizing our society's attitudes about victim blaming. But remember how these attitudes are just old fake news? Yup. No matter your gender, sexual orientation, what you were wearing or what you were doing, *it was never your fault*. I hope that if the #MeToo movement has shown us anything, it is that everyone deserves to be heard and acknowledged when it comes to sexual trauma. That so many people have collectively stepped out from the shadows and shared their stories proves that you are not alone. Speaking out about your trauma does not make you weak, it makes you strong. Sex therapist Vanessa Marin recommends the following mantra when you find yourself minimizing your sexual trauma: "I know it's hard to acknowledge that I've been abused. But it did happen, and it needs my attention. I deserve to acknowledge what happened to me, and to heal."[142]

You might not have control over what happened in your past, but you have 100 per cent ultimate power over your thoughts in this moment. Just let that sink in for a minute. You have a choice right now to run from the past, or to own it. Those scars are beautiful and they make you who you are, but they don't define who you are becoming.

Acknowledging sexual trauma means we must also recognize how these traumas manifest as learned behaviour patterns and self-limiting beliefs. Surviving sexual trauma can often lead to ongoing effects that alter your relationship with your body and impact your relationships with other people. Left unchecked, the effects of sexual trauma can easily bleed into other areas of our lives, and if we have been minimizing the trauma then we may become unaware or have a difficult time coping with these changes. Based upon clients in her sex therapy practice, Marin shares some of the most common behaviour patterns that sexual trauma survivors experience:

- Getting scared or jumpy when approached, talked to, or touched in specific ways.
- Feeling hypervigilant.
- Having a hard time trusting others.
- Feeling scared of losing control.
- Dissociating during sex, feeling like you go somewhere else mentally.
- A low or non-existent sex drive.
- Difficulty getting turned on or reaching orgasm.
- Feeling disconnected from your body, or even hating your body.
- Not knowing how to make healthy and safe decisions about sexual activity.
- Sexual pain conditions and health issues, like vulvodynia (pain during sex) or UTIs.[143]

If any of this sounds familiar to you, and you are a sexual trauma survivor, have you ever tried to connect the dots between what happened to you and how it has impacted your behaviour, sexual body and relationships? Once we begin to acknowledge the trauma, we can make huge strides to reverse the damage that the trauma has caused. Marin recommends making a "trigger list" of the actions and words that make you feel uncomfortable, unsafe or nervous. Because this can be an upsetting and challenging process, she also recommends making a "safe list" of the actions, activities and words that make you feel good and happy. Over time, you may even see the trigger list get shorter and the safe list get longer.

Self-Love and Self-Care

Self-care is more than just a bath bomb in a warm tub surrounded by candles and a glass of wine, or a night at your favourite sports bar playing pinball with the guys. Self-care encompasses the attitude that you take toward yourself, and the practice of compassion and kindness, to yourself. Every day we battle to turn off the inner critic that tells us we're not good enough, not smart enough or not worthy enough. Most of the time, that critic stems from the programmed self-limiting beliefs we were conditioned to accept when we were young. Self-care means truly caring for yourself, body, mind and spirit, and self-love doesn't mean narcissism – it means completely and wholly accepting yourself in the present and embracing your journey to become the best version of yourself in the future.

We do have a tendency as a generation to focus so much on self-love that we can easily abandon people, ideas or goals when they feel like too much effort. But is this really self-love? Or is this just a cop out? Self-love is not about avoiding things that make us uncomfortable. It is about tackling those things head on, knowing that you are your own safe place. Even if something in your life makes you feel triggered, angry or upset, self-love is about having the confidence to know that nothing and nobody can drag you down. You can handle any situation, because you know you are worthy and safe.

But how on earth do we get to that place? Well first of all, we must silence the inner critic. Sometimes, the inner critic's voice is very loud indeed, and other times, when we are in the flow, feeling good and happy and doing what we love, that critic starts to die down (more on flow later on). But in life we can't always do what makes us happy all the time. Sometimes we get stuck in places that make us unhappy, but just because things aren't going how we want, we don't deserve to be subjected to the scalding voice of that inner critic.

There are a few thought exercises that I like to do and that I generally encourage anyone I am working with to follow regularly. The first one is quite simple. Think about your best friend, that one person in your life who is just totally amazing and awesome. Now imagine that friend was going through a hard time or feeling really down. What would you tell them? Would you be their cheerleader and try to cheer them up? I would hope so! Write down a few lines of what you would say to them to help brighten their day.

Now read those words again, only this time, read them to yourself. Feels weird, right? We are all so great at being cheerleaders for the people we love, but few of us have ever really stopped and tried to be cheerleaders for ourselves! Imagine how your best friend would feel if you talked to them in the shitty language of your inner critic. That would not be cool. And if it's not ok to talk to the people you love in that language, why is it ok to speak to yourself like that? The truth is, it's not. Self-love means we are kind to ourselves. Not only with what we put into our bodies, but with the thoughts that we allow to fester in our minds. Overthinking, self-blame and self-judgement destroy our peace of mind, making it harder to heal and grow. Everybody has the right to be their own number one fan and the captain of their own cheerleading team. Having a healthy inner dialogue with yourself doesn't make you an egomaniac or a narcissist. You are allowed to treat yourself kindly, because you deserve it. Everyone does.

The next exercise is one that I've adapted from Julia Cameron's brilliant *The Artist's Way*, which is all about helping people find their creative flow.[144] Think back to a time earlier in your life, where you felt impressionable, confused, powerless or vulnerable. This could be last week, or 15 years ago. It could be the time that sexual trauma happened, or if you're not ready to go there yet, it can be another incident. Think about someone in your life who was there for you, who believed in you, or who supported you. Even if you felt completely alone, I guarantee that there was someone there, because there always is. Now, think about the person who didn't support you, who crushed your dreams or your spirit, or who didn't believe in you. Take out a pen and paper and handwrite (please, handwrite) them each a letter from your present adult self. For the first letter, let the person know how much their belief in you meant. And for the person who made you feel like shit, write them a letter explaining why they were wrong about you. They hurt you, they misjudged you, and here you are a grown adult letting them know that they messed up. When you're done writing, read through what you said, think about how it makes you feel to say those things, and then burn the letters (throwing them in the trash will do, too). Destroying the letters represents your desire to release the feelings of the past. You can do this as many times as you want about as many different people or situations as you choose.

The last exercise is one of my all-time favourites. Where is the place where we are always evaluating ourselves? In front of the mirror, of course! Sadly, no matter how we feel on the inside, many of us do not like to look in the mirror. We see our perceived flaws jumping out at us instead of seeing a gorgeous, complex human being staring back at us. The mirror has no Snapchat filter, no Photoshop, no blurring. It is a pure and unadulterated reflection of us. I strongly believe in reclaiming the mirror as a method for increasing our feelings of self-love. I want you to take a dry-erase marker, a lipstick, an eye shadow pencil or a sticky note, and write on the mirror some of the things you want for yourself: Your goals, your dreams, your intentions, and most importantly, your ideal feelings about yourself. "I am happy," "I deserve success," "I am beautiful" are common ones. You are going to turn your mirror into a vision board of self-love. Write these positive affirmations around your reflection so that when you look at yourself, you actually see all of the good things in your life staring back at you. When I was suffering with health problems, I wrote "I deserve to be healthy" and I stared at that damn scrawl of lipstick every morning until I got better. There were days when just seeing it made me burst into tears, because I felt so far away from where I needed to be. But I kept with it. Maybe this exercise helps reprogramme the brain. Maybe it just makes us feel good to see positive thoughts staring back at us instead of negative ones.

Write in big block letters on the mirror, "I AM ENOUGH" and "I AM WORTHY OF LOVE." If you can, say it out loud to yourself. Yell it out! Scream it at the top of your lungs. But just know that most people can't scream it out at first. I couldn't do it the first time I tried this. I choked the words down into my throat. I've done this exercise with tons of people and most of them have a really hard time saying out loud that they are worthy and enough. It is in direct violation of our inner critic and our self-limiting beliefs, which can create a state of cognitive dissonance when we try to say it aloud. But every time you do say it, it gets easier. You are telling the inner critic to shut the hell up, turning down the volume on the nasty self-limiting beliefs that might be in your head. You are reclaiming your power over yourself and your worthiness of all the good things that are happening and going to happen in your life. Because the truth is, right now, you are enough, and you are worthy of love! Often, the only person in your life who doesn't believe that is you. So today is the day where you get to start believing in *you* and seeing the beauty and greatness that everyone else already sees in you.

Forgiveness

Once we begin the healing process, embracing attitudes of forgiveness can offer us an immensely beneficial pathway to healing and relief. Forgiveness can mean different things to different people, but it usually entails a decision to let go of thoughts of resentment and revenge. Some psychologists argue that true forgiveness at the highest level invokes empathy, compassion and understanding for the person, people or institutions that hurt you. Does forgiveness mean that what happened was ok? No. Does it mean you are letting them "get away" with it? No. I always say that forgiveness does not mean that what happened was ok, it just means you are done shouldering the burden of what happened. You want to release it, to feel free, and to feel ten pounds lighter spiritually. When thoughts of anger and revenge take over our space, they might feel immediately gratifying but over time they will destroy our peace of mind. To paraphrase the Buddha, holding onto anger is like drinking poison and then expecting the other person to die. In reality the poison of anger slowly destroys you from the inside out, never actually reaching the person to whom it has been directed.

Scientific and psychological research has consistently demonstrated the vital benefits of practising forgiveness for our physical and psychological health. People who learn to forgive tend to have healthier relationships, reductions of chronic stress and anxiety,[145] fewer symptoms of depression, reduction in "toxic" anger, improved self-esteem and improved mental health overall.[146] The mind–body connection is so incredible that people who learn forgiveness training also reap a host of physical health benefits, including a reduction in blood pressur,[147] better outcomes for heart health[148] and even a strengthened immune system.

Why all of the benefits? According to the experts, forgiveness offers a significant reduction in the chronic stressors that burden us, which explains its robust effects on reducing psychological distress and enhancing wellbeing. It frees us up and helps to quiet that inner critic a little bit more. Dr Bob Enright, who pioneered the study of the psychology of forgiveness more than three decades ago, also believes that the magic of forgiveness lies in its ability to help us reduce what he calls "toxic" anger. He asserts that "There's nothing wrong with healthy anger, but when anger is very deep and long lasting, it can do a number on us systemically. When you get rid of anger, your muscles relax, you're less anxious, you have more energy, your immune system can strengthen."[149]

Furthermore, forgiveness can actually help us build self-esteem by reframing the way in which we see ourselves. According to Enright, "When people are beaten down by injustice, you know who they end up not liking? Themselves. When you stand up to the pain of what happened to you and offer goodness to the person who hurt you, you change your view of yourself."[150] When we forgive, we begin to see ourselves as brave, compassionate survivors instead of victims of other people's actions.

This all sounds great, but how can we bring these ideas into action? There are several models of forgiveness training, including Enright's 20-step model which focuses on four stages: Uncovering one's negative feelings about the offence; deciding to forgive; working toward understanding the offending person; and discovering empathy and compassion for them. Worthington's REACH model offers a five-step plan: Recalling the hurt; empathizing with your partner; giving altruistic gifts; committing to changing attitudes; and holding onto forgiveness. A review of 54 studies on the efficacy of these models showed that both were found to be effective for helping people forgive and also for improving their mental health.[151]

If forgiveness feels like something you want to work on, and/ or something you believe you might benefit from, I encourage you to review links to forgiveness therapy training resources in the recommended reading section. As Enright says, "Without our deserving it, we can experience thunderous injustices. The injury was unfair, the person who created it was unfair. But now we have a place for healing."[152]

Flow

The final step to healing from old social conditioning and living empowered lives involves bringing ourselves into a state of flow. What is flow, exactly? Flow is a state of optimal consciousness where we feel our best and perform our best. According to Dr Mikhal Csikszentmihalyi, hailed as the originator of the concept in positive psychology, "Flow" is a state of:

Being completely involved in an activity for its own sake. The ego falls away. Time flies. Every action, movement, and thought follows inevitably from the previous one, like playing jazz. Your whole being is involved, and you're using your skills to the utmost.[153]

According to Csikszentmihalyi's groundbreaking work, the feeling of flow is associated with these ten factors, although not all of them have to be present in order to experience flow. Have you ever experienced some or all of these?

1 You feel a complete focus of attention.
2 The activity is intrinsically rewarding.
3 You have clear, attainable (although still challenging) goals.
4 You have a feeling of peace and losing yourself.
5 There is an element of timelessness, or, losing track of time during the activity.
6 You receive immediate feedback.
7 You know that the task is doable, and you can strike a balance between skill level and the challenge presented.
8 You feel a sense of personal control over your efforts.
9 You lose track of your physical needs.
10 You experience an unusually high level of concentration.[154]

There are two reasons why I feel that cultivating flow is essential for our healing processes. First, when we are confused, traumatized, holding onto anger and feeling hurt, experiencing extra noise going on in our brains and much tension in our bodies, it can be challenging to access flow. While some artists do claim to thrive off their pain and use it for their creative expression, there is a difference between channelling your pain into a creative outlet and being so wrapped up in your pain that you can't concentrate or focus. That difference? Flow! When we are hurting, we actually need the relief that comes with flow, the calmness that it brings us, the pleasure and passion we experience, the joy it triggers deep inside, and the creativity and productivity that can ensue.

Second, when it comes to healing from sexual trauma, remember that sexual energy symbolizes the flow energy of the universe. If you've ever had a dream about giving birth, you might have realized that this is not necessarily literal, but usually reflects a time of birthing your creative energy into the world. Remember, sex is the ultimate creator, it creates life! So, when our sexual energy is all locked up, it would make sense that our ability to get into flow would feel blocked. The shamans used to say, about tribal dance, "Free the feet to free the head" and I believe the adage also applies here. Free the head by losing our heads in flow. Ha! Sometimes, we just need to focus on our flow and allow it to facilitate healing to take place in our mind and body.

One of the coolest things about flow is that it actually changes our brain functioning and neurochemistry, literally making us feel happier. A variety of processes occur simultaneously in the brain when we enter a state of flow: Brain wave transitions, prefrontal cortex deactivation and neurochemical changes. Together they help explain why during flow, the brain is capable of enhanced creativity and productivity.

Brain Wave Transitions. While in a state of flow, our brainwaves transition from the more rapid beta waves we experience during waking consciousness and everyday activities to slower alpha waves (associated with relaxed and effortless alertness, peak performance and creativity) and even much slower theta waves (associated with the deeper dream-state consciousness).

Pre-Frontal Cortex Deactivation (PFC). The PFC is the area of the brain that houses higher-level cognitions, including those that help us to cultivate our ego and sense of self. During a flow state this area becomes deactivated, helping us lose ourselves in the task at hand and silence our inner critics, fears and self-doubts.

Neurochemistry. Flow states also trigger a release of many of the pleasurable and performance inducing chemicals in the brain, including dopamine, serotonin, norepinephrine and endorphins. A 2014 study published in the journal *Neuron* showed that when we are intrinsically curious about an outcome and driven for answers, dopamine is released in the brain, helping to solidify our memories. These findings suggest why flow states are good for promoting learning and memory in addition to creativity.[155]

Sounds wonderful right? Can you recall the last time you were in a state of flow? I get there sometimes when I am writing. I lose time and suddenly three hours have gone by and I've written 20 pages without really remembering what happened. I used to think I was channelling some otherworldly being (or something?), but now I know that I'm just in a state of focused flow. My brainwaves change and my brain gets flooded with happy chemicals. I come out of a flow state feeling relaxed and happy, instead of stressed out or angry. People can find flow states anywhere and everywhere: Snowboarding, knitting, yoga, running, painting, playing sports, playing musical instruments, composing, computer coding, dancing, hooping, poi spinning, hiking, swimming, cooking, doing calculus (yes, really!) and so on.

Are you connected to what makes you flow? Do you want to bring more flow into your life? Based on my experiences with flow, I offer these eight steps as a pathway for opening yourself up to this wondrous potential:

1 *Do Something that Interests You*
Flow comes most naturally when we are intrinsically motivated, excited and curious about the task. So, if you are looking to get creative and productive, choose to focus on a task that you enjoy and feel passionate about. If this is for work, or you don't have a choice of the task, try to identify elements of the task that excite you. Maybe there are certain parts of a project or elements of an assignment that interest you? Pay special attention to those. If you're not sure what interests you, turn off the phone/Internet and go try new things until you find something that clicks!

2 *Set Clear Goals*
Be specific when you are getting started on a task. What is the goal you are aiming for? Are you trying to finish a painting? Write a new song? Complete a presentation? Or perfect a new yoga pose? This will help to hone your focus and keep you on task. If you try to do too much at once it could overwhelm you, and if you do too little you might not spend enough time in deep concentration to reach a flow state. Knowing how to set your goals is all about practice and balance.

3 *Find a Quiet and Productive Time*
Most people find that an environment of peace and quiet works best for inducing a state of flow, possibly because of how brainwave patterns shift into slower frequencies during flow. When you begin your work, try to cultivate a calm, quiet environment. Also, make sure to identify when you are most productive: For some, this is first thing in the morning, and for others it is afternoon. For me, it is late at night. Identify the right time for you to be creative and block it off to engage in your flow time. It is worth taking the time to make flow happen, even if it's impinging on your Netflix and chill time. Just go for it!

4 *Avoid Interruptions and Distractions*
Interruptions are the enemy of flow. Every time we get distracted, whether it is a roommate speaking to us, our phone beeping, emails coming in, a distracting song or a messy desk, it can pull us out of flow and quicken our brainwaves back to beta state. When you decide it is time to get into flow, turn off the phone, ask your friends, family or roommates not to disturb you, and tidy up your space before you get started. Let me just say it again, with emphasis: TURN. OFF. THE. PHONE! No Snapchat or IG allowed ever when you're doing your flow thing. Social media is literally the anthesis of flow. If you're in the art studio, organize and clean your brushes. If you're in the gym, clean up any stray equipment or articles of clothing. If you're going surfing, get your board all nice and waxed and your wet suit cleaned. This helps set the intention and prime your brain for what you're about to do.

5 *Focus for as Long as You Can*
Once you are able to sit down during a quiet productive time without distractions, try to stay focused for as long as you can. At first, especially if you are new to the task, you may only be able to focus for five or ten minutes. This is ok: Just keep practising! Sometimes if you lose the flow, taking a break can help. I keep my yoga wheel, mat and bolster in my office on the ground right next to my desk. When I begin to lose focus, I stop writing and start doing yoga and stretches until I feel more at ease. Find the thing that works for you. As you continue to direct your energies into focusing, you will train your brain to more easily and fluidly drop into the flow state and before long, hours will be passing by like minutes.

6 *Match Your Skills to the Task*
We can best enter flow when we are working on a task that is suited to our skill level. In other words, when we are well prepared for the task at hand, we are more likely to experience flow. Csikszentmihalyi gives the example of a

runner experiencing flow during a marathon for which she has trained for several months. Or consider a skilled graphic artist drawing the designs for her new comic book. But remember, you don't have to be really good at something to get into flow! You just have to be aware of what kinds of tasks you can actually complete. So, if you're new at guitar, you can still get into flow practising that G chord over and over until it sounds perfect.

7   *But There Is No Harm in Stretching Your Skills Slightly*
Your skills should match the task at hand, but it is also possible to stretch your skills slightly past your comfort zone to maximize flow. A little bit of a challenge can be a great thing. Try a new yoga move that is extra difficult or record a song using new software. As long as the background skills are there, pushing yourself a little bit can be excellent for bringing you into a concentrated, productive state. I think about learning to ski, and how I was afraid to go down the blues because I had only ever done green runs. But when I did finally go down that blue run, I was so incredibly focused that the whole run flew by and I felt like that challenge was just what I needed to get into flow.

8   *Emphasize Process, Not Outcome*
Finally, please remember that the experience of flow is a *process* not an outcome. In other words, working and creating from a place of flow is a life skill that you can strive to master with practice, and this usually does not happen overnight. Just keep trying and do not give up even if you don't nail it right away. Remember, flow is all about *enjoyment* and living in the *present moment.* If you become too wrapped up in the outcome, then it can take your enjoyment away (much like orgasms!). Who really cares what the painting looks like, so long as you enjoyed painting it, right!? Flow and the quest to get into flow should feel like a pressure-free experience. The second we put pressure on ourselves, that inner critic can rear its ugly head and sabotage us. Just keep trying and continue

to be open to the endless stream of untapped creativity always flowing through you. You can do this!

I hope that this chapter has helped empower you as you continue your sex positive journey. Remember, you are normal, you are worthy of love and you are enough!!!! Take this self-knowledge and spread it like wildfire. And as we continue to change the world, we must not forget to continue to work on ourselves. As my idol Carl Jung famously said,

> *Your vision will become clear only when you can look into your own heart ... Who looks outside, dreams; Who looks inside, awakens.*[156]

And that's what we need to heal ourselves, and it is also what the world needs right now: Dreams and awakening. We need to dream BIG as we continue to rewrite the script about love and shred the institutions that no longer serve us. But in order to rebuild and grow, we need to awaken to our own power, becoming aware of how our programmed self-limiting beliefs might be holding us back, so that we can become unstoppable and build a future that reflects the best parts of who we are becoming. And no (wo)man is an island, so a huge part of that future we are creating involves our relationships with other people. How do we integrate our newfound abilities to cope with our personal shifting attitudes to maximize our relationship satisfaction and happiness? It starts with the right partner.

PART THREE
REDEFINING OUR RELATIONSHIPS

CHAPTER 7
RIGHT PARTNER, RIGHT RELATIONSHIP

In spite of the difficulties and challenges many of us face when it comes to relating, deep down, most of us just want to be loved and to build deep connections with other humans. If we are truly seeking to build sex positive relationships, we must do so with a partner who respects our mutual freedom to be ourselves and to love how we choose. In the context of a generation that does more "chatting online" than dating and possibly does more orgasming alone than with a partner, can we really blame ourselves for not knowing where to start when it comes to finding the right partner(s)?

Now, remember, the idea of the "right partner" is entirely subjective. You might be looking for the right partner for a long-term relationship, or the right person just for tonight. Heck, you might even be looking for the right partner for a new "textlationship" (more on those later on). Perhaps you're looking for the right partner to jump down the rabbit hole of experimentation with you, from anything to polyamory to bondage. You might be looking for your first pansexual connection. Maybe you don't know what you want, but you know what you don't want. Perhaps you've been ghosted in the past, and you're looking for someone who is upfront and honest. You might already be attached and looking to see if you're with a person who shares your goals. You might be currently single and want to remain that way, but you know this information might come in handy in the future. In this chapter I'm going to share some of my favourite psychological theories, models and research about relationships to help lay the foundations for building sex positive relationships.

Power Couple or Bust? The Jay-Z and Beyoncé Effect

But first, let's take stock of our goals when it comes to love and relationships. A 2018 interview with therapists who treat millennial patients revealed that many of us are looking for a partner who can fulfil *all* of our needs: a best friend who is also a financial equal, as well an erotic match and potentially one day, a strong co-parent. Coined the *"Jay-Z and Beyoncé effect"*, the new standard for relationships appears to be *power couple or bust*!

The phrase *"power couple"* was even added to the *Oxford English Dictionary* (OED) in 2016, referring to two ambitious people with powerful careers in a domestic partnership or a marriage.[157] It stands out as one of the few two-word entries in the OED, and it appears we can thank the increasing popularity of the cult of celebrity for making us believe that this is an attainable, desirable option to reach for. Why is the power couple goal so appealing to many of us? Perhaps it is because the idea of the power couple goes against the traditional gender norms of the man as the provider or breadwinner and the woman as the homemaker. Given our tendencies to disrupt the norms surrounding sex and gender, it makes sense that we would love the idea of a relationship that alludes to the commitment of marriage, tucked safely away in the context of both parties' mutual independence. If both members of a power couple are successful on their own, then perhaps they are married for love and respect rather than for financial necessity. Does that make the marriage somehow better, safer or more meaningful?

Or perhaps the "power couple" notion has become more popular lately because we want to find that partner with whom we can grow. Women have traditionally had their careers cut short by a patriarchal society that for the last century has emphasized child rearing over career. Equally important in the rejection of traditional gender norms is millennial women's waning enthusiasm about being responsible for all of the housework, child rearing and chores. Women now want to see an equal division of labour on the home front. They also want their needs to be met regarding sex, emphasizing a desire for true intimacy.

With all of these needs, from household equality, to deep sexual intimacy, to independent commitment, to finding someone who really inspires you, to both being independently successful, it is hardly surprising that a lot of us feel like there must be something inherently "wrong" with us because we have such a hard time finding a lasting commitment with someone who meets these extensive relationship criteria. In fact, this is a theme that consistently emerges in therapy with millennials: The feeling that we are just not good enough or that there must be something wrong with us because we can't seem to get everything we want out of life. A report on the top relationship problems millennials faced according to therapists recently revealed these six questions as the most commonly asked (can you relate to them?):

1 Is there someone better out there for me?
2 What is the point of getting married?
3 What does this text from my crush or partner mean?
4 Why am I not dating anyone?
5 I don't want to be financially tied down to my partner!
6 I'm ready for the next stage of life. My partner needs to grow up![158]

We all want to know that a strong connection is possible, because sometimes it can seem like we will never find our Prince or Princess Charming. Again, part of the problem here is that what we perceive on social media regarding all of these happy power couples does not actually reflect their real lives, thanks to the joys of Internet identity management and people's desire to post positive, inspiring content to generate likes and followers. Seeing so many fit, happy, successful people on social media posting their epic vacations and living their perfect lives can really crush your self-esteem and make you feel totally inadequate, or like a failure in love. But do not fret! The right person is out there, but you might have to make slight sacrifices or date someone outside of the box. If you're single, try expanding your horizons to someone you wouldn't typically date and see what happens. Or, stay single and enjoy your freedom and independence. Keep building your career and when things are going well that right person may appear who is on the exact same path as you are!

The Five Love Languages

One of the most useful tools I have encountered in my work as a social psychologist is Gary Chapman's *The Five Love Languages*.[159] This model has helped me tremendously to build a better understanding with all of the people I relate with, romantic as well as family and friends. While entire books have been written on the subject (and I encourage you to explore them), I want to briefly summarize and explain how using this model can benefit feelings of validation in your relationship and enhance your ability to communicate with your partner – something, in my opinion, that many of us lack due to our obsession with communicating primarily via technology (more on that in chapter 9!).

According to Chapman's (1992) book, people express love in different ways, and feel loved and appreciated in different contexts.[160] These are our "*love languages*" and they vary from person to person. The way we express our love is learned and conditioned from the ways that our partners and families express their love, as well as from our own individual personality types and past experiences. When we can understand and decode our partner's love language, it can take a lot of the confusion and guesswork out of their expectations and their needs. The five love languages are: Words of Affirmation, Acts of Service, Receiving Gifts, Quality Time and Physical Touch. Most people have a primary love language, as well as a secondary love language. In the recommended reading section I have included a link to quizzes so that you can determine your primary and secondary love language as well as that of any potential partners. Most likely you will be able to tell from reading the following description which model best describes how you give and receive love:

- *Words of Affirmation*: If this is your love language, you express and receive love through words and phrases that build people up, like simple compliments and acknowledgements. This isn't about being insecure and needing to be complimented or told "I love you" just to feel safe and adequate. Rather, people with this love language appreciate being recognized because it shows how their partner is actively thinking about them and noticing the little things. Conversely, people who have words of affirmation as their love language will also feel more deeply hurt and take a longer time to forgive when negative or insulting things are said to them. Even if a comment means little to you, remember that those words and comments mean quite a lot more to your partner.
- *Acts of Service:* The motto of this love language is that "actions speak louder than words." A person with this love language shows their love by doing chores and other activities that lessen their partner's load, like cooking a meal, doing the laundry or cleaning the back yard. These are often selfless acts that are designed to show love through the sacrifice and quiet effort entailed. Note that if this is your partner's love language, then doing these tasks to show your love to them out of a sense of obligation or with a negative

begrudging attitude will not be interpreted as "love". These actions must be undertaken with a sense of positivity and joy that you are bringing them happiness!

- *Receiving Gifts:* Gifts as a love language is an interesting one because people often associate it with materialism, gold digging or money grabbing. However, receiving gifts as a love language has less to do with the lavishness of the gifts and more to do with their thoughtfulness. Meaningful and thoughtful gifts show your partner that you appreciate and think of them. This can be something super small, from picking up their favourite desert as a treat, to surprising them with a copy of a magazine with their favourite singer on the cover. But if this is your partner's love language and you don't think gifting is important, they may end up feeling invalidated and unloved.

- *Quality Time:* People whose love language is quality time are all about their partner giving them undivided attention, without phones, work or other distractions. This lets them know that they are important and loved because their partner is willing to forsake everything else going on to spend an intimate one-on-one moment with them. Of course, snuggling up for some Netflix and chill is still an option for quality time, because this is something that the two of you are doing together. If your partner's love language is quality time, every time you cancel a date or you aren't present for your time together, they may feel unloved or neglected.

- *Physical Touch:* People whose love language is physical touch long for some type of sustained physical contact to reinforce the bonds in their relationship. People wrongly assume that the level of touch has to be sexual or intimate for a person to feel satisfied, but that is not the case. Rather, the touch in question can involve holding hands, hugging, snuggling, massaging or just a hand on your knee or shoulders. If your partner's primary love language is physical touch, then without it they will feel unloved, no matter how many gifts you give, affirmations you offer, or acts of service you perform.

I want you to think back to your last serious relationship. If you are in one right now, even better. (If you've never been in one, this exercise also works by thinking about a family member or friend.) Think about the way that your partner shows you love: Do they often do the dishes or buy you gifts? Do they frequently say nice things to you? Do they touch you and hold your hand regularly? Or do they plan special dates and activities where the two of you can be alone?

The way a person shows their love is reflective of the way that they seek to receive love. Essentially, they are acting out their love language, showing you what *they* respond to, how they want you to better love *them*. Thinking back to your most recent relationship, were you able to show them love in the same way that they showed you love? Or did you show them love in the way that you expected and desired to receive love?

Let me give you a personal example. I am (not surprisingly) very much a physical touch person. This is my primary love language and I'd say that quality time is my secondary. When I was living with my primary partner many years ago, I would try to lie on his chest while we were snuggling up for some sex on the sofa, and he'd literally recoil. I'd grab his hand and he would pull it away. After a while, I became so distraught I honestly believed that he did not love me, because he seemed to have no interest in physical touch. And because he wasn't loving me in the language that I expected, I could not receive his love.

His love language? Acts of service with words of affirmation secondary. To this day he's still running around the house fixing everything, preparing gourmet meals and constantly coming up with organizational scenarios that make my (messy) life easier. When we first got together, I did not know about the love languages and I didn't even notice that he was showing me his love in a different language, one that I could not understand because I thought my language was the *only* language.

After dating for a few months, when I finally approached him with the usual accusatory words of "YOU DON'T LOVE ME!" and explained why I felt this way, he shared with me that he had been experiencing extreme nerve sensitivity, making physical touch in some areas of his body (especially his chest which is where I was always trying to place my head) incredibly uncomfortable. He also told me, "Of course I love you, baby, look at everything I'm always doing around the house to make your life easier!" At that point, I realized that I had never really acknowledged that he was doing these things to show his love. Before that, I always thought that he should show his love by letting me bury my head in his chest and lie there all night long.

At this point I began researching the expectations of loving and I stumbled upon *The Five Love Languages*. Once we realized that we had completely different love languages and understood why we both often felt invalidated and unloved by the other's language, we were able to work on rebuilding our intimacy. He made efforts to engage in physical touch on parts of his body that didn't hurt, and when we were watching TV, he'd grab my leg and place his hand there, knowing that it mattered to me. And I began putting more effort into taking care of things around the house and thanking him for his efforts, since his secondary language was words of affirmation. We're not perfect by any means but this model has really allowed us to continue to cohabit and grow together, and I hope it might do the same for you.

Karmic Relationships

From a spiritual perspective, karma refers to the accumulation of every thought, intention and action from this current lifetime and all our previous lifetimes. Now whether you believe in karma, past lives, reincarnation, the human soul energy, and so on, the concept of "karmic" relationship is still inherently valuable because it reflects how the ways we have learned to relate, and the ways we have acted in those relationships, will continue to shape the relationships in our present and future. From this perspective, every single relationship we enter has a significance to our life's journey and to our personal development. In fact, maybe every person with whom we connect serves as a reflection of inner ourselves, and of our deeply rooted subconscious struggles, conditioning and issues. Ever heard the phrase "a reason, a season, a lifetime" when it comes to describing relationships? In this sense, there is always a lesson to be learned from every relationship, and the more we can do the inner work to connect to ourselves and discover that lesson, the more we will be able to grow and to pursue relationships that are more deeply soulful and satisfying (a process I like to call "*levelling up*").

In her book *The Karma Queens' Guide to Relationships*, Dr Carmen Harra speculates that there are four types of relationships we find ourselves in throughout our lives.[161] Whether you believe in karma or not, it is hard to argue that we choose our partners for a reason, and that this reason embodies the totality of our life experiences when it comes to love, loss and personal growth. This perspective may offer you insight into the type of relationship you are in now (if you are in one), and the types of partners you might seek to find in your future.

1 *Compromise Relationships*: In Dr Harra's experiences as a
   counsellor, she found these to be the common types of
   relationships (accounting for roughly 70 per cent of all
   relationships). People often settle with each other for the
   wrong reasons but become comfortable because they have
   children, the same home, shared bank accounts and so
   on, making them afraid to walk away from the marriage
   or relationship. These relationships can easily become
   dysfunctional or toxic over time because there is not
   enough real love and the other pragmatic reasons are not
   good enough to make the marriage succeed and grow. Are

compromise relationships still the most common type of relationships for millennials, who are much less likely to get married, especially for reasons of practicality?

2 *Transitory Relationships*: These relationships are short, reflecting what people do during life transitions: We like to play the field! These can often be rebound relationships that happen after people leave more serious relationships, reflecting a specific set of circumstances in a person's life rather than a deep soul connection. Transitory relationships tend to be more superficial and less commitment oriented and usually do not entail a serious investment of energy or resources. My advice with these types of relationships? Be honest with yourself if you are in this stage. If this is your semester abroad in Greece before you go back to Berkeley to finish your degree, then Dimitri is probably not your soul mate. Trying to hold on and make this permanent will only delay your personal evolution and lead to feelings of resentment and unhappiness.

3 *Karmic Relationships*: Have you ever met someone and out of the blue felt an extremely strong attraction to them, almost like déjà-vu? A type of feeling that you cannot explain, one that you don't want to pursue but you are so drawn to them you have no choice but to explore it? When we meet someone like this, it reflects a truly karmic relationship in this life (or from our previous lives, if you believe in that sort of thing). This person appears to help teach you an important lesson. And once that karma is resolved, the door to this relationship closes and there will be no need to look back. Karmic relationships are sudden, quick and end abruptly once their purpose has been identified. How do we find out the purpose? When we do the inner work to understand why the attraction is so strong, the lesson will be revealed.

4 *Soul Mate Relationships:* The rarest and most beautiful relationship, Dr Harra predicts that up to 10 per cent of all

relationships are soul mate relationships. These are intense pairings, where two people become so mentally inseparable that they cannot bear to be apart, but in a different sense from people who are co-dependent. We will talk more a little bit later in the chapter about where the idea of "soul mates" actually comes from and how it offers relevancy to our dating worlds today.[162]

The Triangle Theory of Love

Let's say you are in a relationship, and you know it is not a toxic relationship, but you are not sure if you're on the same page as your partner. Perhaps you are in a brand new relationship. Maybe you just started talking after meeting on Tinder or you've been on a few dates after getting hooked up by friends and you're wondering if this is the real deal or not. Relationship psychologists have typically postulated that a romantic relationship is comprised of three components: Intimacy, passion and commitment. Intimacy reflects your closeness and attachment to each other. Passion reflects the excitement you have for each other in and out of the bedroom, and commitment reflects, well, the dreaded C word for many of us, the intention and the decision to stick together.

Psychologist Robert Sternberg developed the "Triangle Theory of Love" (1986) by placing each of these three constructs as points on a triangle then defining different types of love by the balance of these three elements. How does the geometry of your relationship look, and would it match the one that your partner drew? One exercise involves asking couples to draw out how they thought their triangles looked, and the closer the match, the greater the likelihood of relationship satisfaction. If you're currently in a relationship, think about what your triangle might look like: Where is your balance of intimacy, passion and commitment?[163]

How close you feel, how much passion you have, and how much commitment you intend determines the type of relationship you will have. Sternberg details eight types of relationships based upon the triangle theory. Which one(s) are you in now, and which have you had in the past?

1 *Non-Love:* This is the absence of intimacy, passion and commitment. Basically, no triangle.
2 *Liking/Friendship*: Intimacy only, meaning you share feelings of closeness and bondedness but no passion or commitment. Sometimes people in a "textlationship" who chat a lot online or via text end up in this realm.
3 *Infatuation*: Passion only, sometimes called "puppy love" or lust, and a good reflection of many of the hookups that stem from online dating. People are attracted to each other but aren't especially close and have little desire to commit. Often intimacy builds over time and this can turn into romantic love or consummate love. If the other two parts of the triangle don't develop, this will fizzle out pretty quickly.
4 *Empty Love*: Commitment only, with no intimacy or passion. Ugh, this is our worst nightmare and depicts many of our parents' marriages, akin to the *compromise* relationships discussed in the previous section.
5 *Romantic Love*: In this case, we have passion and intimacy, but no commitment. Definitely reflective of much of the millennial relationship landscape, these could be one-night stands or hookups, or just two people who really want to maintain their independence.
6 *Fatuous Love:* When we have passion and commitment, but no real closeness. This makes me think of people who meet each other in Vegas on a night out and get married at the Elvis Chapel the next day. They're all swept off their feet, but they really don't "know" each other at all.
7 *Companionate Love:* When we have intimacy and commitment but no passion, we are usually looking at family members or super close friends who have vowed to stay in each other's lives. There isn't any sexual excitement

or drive here. Sometimes, people in long-term relationships end up here when the spark starts to fade. Did you ever make a pact with your gay best friend that you'd get married by the age of 35 if you never found anyone? That's another picture of companionate love.

8 *Consummate Love:* The centre of the triangle, consummate love reflects the ideal or "perfect couple" love where there is intimacy, passion and commitment. Of course, this is often harder to maintain than it is to create, as life throws us curve balls and our feelings of passion can wane into companionate love. While this was the "ideal" when Sternberg wrote the theory, is this still the ideal for us today?

Coping with the New Relationship Energy

The NRE, or, New Relationship Energy, is a psychological and physiological drive state we experience at the beginning of most sexual and romantic relationships that is characterized by giddiness, excitement and that "rosy glow" of being in love. Baumeister (1999) has argued that passion is a function of changes in intimacy over time, such that rising intimacy will create a strong feeling of passion.[164] As we rapidly become close and intimate, we feel very much in love. Cue the turtle dove staring at each other from across the room, constant text messages of heart-faced emojis (and dick pics) and using words like "destiny", "soul mate" and "forever". Of course, like all good things, this "honey moon period" usually fades in a couple of months. For people in many types of relationships (including monogamous as well as non-monogamous, discussed in the next chapter), the occurrence of the NRE is not necessarily a bad thing. The NRE can feel absolutely amazing for the people experiencing it, but please, don't jump into important life decisions like buying a house, or a car, or introducing your kids (if you have kids). In these early phases, you don't know for certain if you're just high on love drugs in your brain, or if this is the real thing.

Two Halves: "How Do I Find My Soul Mate?"

Guess how many sex workshops I've done where the first thing that my audience members ask me at the end is, "How do I find my soul mate?" or "How do I know when I've found my soul mate?" It's a lot. It's happened so many times in fact that I wanted to include it in this chapter, because a "soul mate" in the esoteric/energetic/spiritual sense is pretty different from a soul mate in the Disney sense, and I'm never exactly sure which one people are talking about.

If you feel like consummate love is the relationship goal for which you are striving, then you've probably also considered the idea of a soul mate as something that sounds appealing. Many people have. We can blame Disney and its whole "princess gets rescued by a prince" narrative for programming our subconscious into believing that there is only one true person out there for us. Of course, as we will learn in the next chapter, some of us completely reject the notion of one person altogether.

Many of us believe that a soul mate is someone we were destined to find, our perfect match, our one true love. Others believe that a soul mate is someone with whom we share a karmic connection, or someone with whom through past lives we are intimately bonded. Others would say that we can have multiple soul mates, but only one twin flame (more on that later). I believe that what you think your soul mate relationship should resemble will determine whether you believe you've found them or not. In other words, there is no "right" or "wrong" soul mate, no definitive way to know for sure if you've found them. It's a decision, a feeling, an intuition, whatever you want to call it.

To help you decide what your soul mate relationship should look and feel like, I thought it would be valuable here to discuss some of the perspectives on soul mate and twin flame relationships. Please note this perspective comes via the esoteric/energy traditions more than from psychology.

Finding a Soul Mate

Elizabeth Gilbert (author of *Eat, Pray, Love*) has talked extensively about soul mates. On Oprah's Super Soul Sunday in 2014, she explained that while everyone thinks your soul mate is a perfect match, your one true fit,

> a true soul mate is a mirror, the person who shows you everything that's holding you back, the person who brings you to your own attention so you can change your life. A true soul mate is probably the most important person you will ever meet, because they tear down your walls and smack you awake.[165]

I love this definition because it serves as an allegory for everything our generation is doing when it comes to love, sex and relationships: Tearing down the rotting old structures and replacing them with something more authentic. Of course, when it comes to interpersonal relationships, soul mate relationships demand a certain level of vulnerability to criticism, owning our mistakes and cultivating a willingness to change, which can be daunting even for the best of us. Gilbert even highlights how sometimes people have to leave because the relationship is just too intense. Despite what we might assume about soul mates being "forever" relationships, this is not always the case. Sometimes, when the lessons have been learned or we have weathered the rough patch, it is time to move on.

Anaiya Sophia, kundalini yoga teacher and certified Priestess of the Rose Line of the Grail Lineage (yes, really!), uniquely defines the differences between a soul family, a soul mate and a twin flame. Take it with a grain of salt, believe it, or leave it altogether, this perspective could be useful for many of us who see sexuality as a spiritual experience.

According to Sophia's perspective, twin flames are "forged from the fires of creation at the very same time and left to cool entwined around each other" for eons, until there is movement and they are forced to separate in opposite directions.[166] She writes about how suffering besets twin flames during their separation, which can last many lifetimes, and the twin flame reunion can feel painful as the two soul halves are reminded of their sadness and loss at their journeys spent apart. Twin flames must overcome their fear of losing each other again before they can enter into a sacred union. Their love is steadfast and enduring, eternal and continues long after their experience in this human body.

Wow! That sounds pretty intense to me! According to Sophia, in addition to our one twin flame who is both our polar opposite but also literally shares our soul, we also have 12 soul mates, created close to us at the time of the original creation of our souls. She believes that six will be male, six will be female, and that each one will carry the energetic signature of one of the 12 houses of the zodiac and their 12 associated planets. She explains, "the purpose of meeting and engaging with soul mates is to create a two-way relationship that refines, sculpts, and shapes the other individual into becoming more of themselves," basically readying and strengthening us for our twin soul reunion.[167] She alludes to similar themes as mentioned previously, including an instant recognition when we meet our soul mates, and how it can often feel like looking in a mirror. Soul mates can be romantic or friendly, we often just love everything about them! But we don't have the same desires to literally merge our souls with them that we do with our one twin flame.

Sophia also uses the flower of life geometry to explain how we have 12 soul mates and 144 soul family members (these are our soul mates' soul mates). We talk a lot in the spiritual context about finding our "soul family" and how we feel much more at home around them than our physical families. Maybe you can relate? When I first read *Sacred Sexual Union*, I spent a while thinking about who my 12 soul mates could be? Have I met them yet? Which signs of the zodiac were they? What about my soul family? I don't have answers to any of these questions, but they have sure made me think. Maybe by planting these ideas into your consciousness to marinate for a while, they might one day have meaning for you, too.

Features of Sex Positive Relationships

All of this talk about soul mates and that perfect match might feel authentic for some of us, but these ideas could also be reflections of the fake news conditioning that has programmed our minds for too long. I could go on and on about the number of films, books and magazines (even comic books!) that continue to reinforce the idea of one "true" mate for each of us (and I'm sure you can come up with plenty of examples yourself). But as we'll see in the next chapter, some of us feel the most comfortable with multiple partners and multiple loves. I share all of this content on soul mates because I am frequently asked about it (especially from a spiritual point of view), but I also caution anyone from seeking it out or ascribing to it so completely that it reduces your options or makes you feel unsatisfied.

Maybe instead of soul mate relationships, we should be looking for truly *Sex Positive* relationships, which can feel much more fluid and adaptive than the idea of the one true mate. I believe that in a sex positive relationship, you can:

- Be whoever you want sexually.
- Do whatever you want sexually (so long as you are not causing harm without consent).
- Never have to apologize for your sexual identity or expression.
- Love your body and your partner(s) body/bodies unconditionally.
- Know that your sexual decision-making is valid because it belongs to YOU.
- Feel supported by your partner(s) without shame, guilt or ridicule for your sexual expression.

- Openly communicate about experimentation, kink and other sexual innovations.
- Feel comfortable enough to be truly *honest* about who you are.
- Work through sexual trauma together in a healthy way.

If this sounds like it is right for you, then read on as we explore how the new styles of relationships are emphasizing fluidity, consent and freedom.

CHAPTER 8

RELATIONSHIP FLUIDITY

In addition to rejecting outdated stereotypes, redefining gender, integrating technology, becoming more spiritual and reclaiming orgasm, another way that people are radically redefining love and sex in this new era involves changing how we regard monogamy and committed relationships. People are embracing fluid styles of relating which have less to do with traditional norms and more to do with the authentic ways that they feel. In this chapter, we will explore how some people are monogamous, and other people may fluctuate in their relationship styles as they become exposed to new ideas, partners and changes within themselves. A huge part of my personal journey has been moving past the notion that the one man/one woman couple is the only acceptable way to live your life. By now you already know that when it comes to love and sex, words like moral, normal and right serve more as subjective value judgements than as accurate scientific fact!

And yet, many people are made to feel like failures, or just bad human beings, because we struggle with fidelity or with staying sexually turned on or active with only one partner. For many, monogamy has been staged like a set-up where failure is the only option. Think about it like this: You can be faithful and happily married for 30 years, but if you mess up – even only *one time* – then according to some accounts, you have failed in your marriage. You have failed your partner, your family, your religion and/or your community. The pressure exerted by this extreme standard of perfection is in my opinion not only part of what drives so many people to secretly cheat, but also what drives the divorce rates in our society sky high.

What if there was another way to find happiness in committed relationships? A way to be completely open and honest with your partner, and to experiment in a safe environment where both parties gave consent? Instead of secretly cheating out of fear and pressure that your relationship will end, what if you could communicate about your desires and learn to share these sexual experiences without possession, rage or jealousy? Ten years ago, I would not have believed it, but during the past several years I have discovered a new type of relationship that I never even knew was possible. No matter the label, the best relationship is one where all partners get to set their own parameters and stick to them in a way that makes them feel supported, validated, and hopefully, super turned on.

People in Relationships Often Cheat

Like many of the fake old news paradigms pertaining to love and sex (homophobia, transphobia, Victorian era standards, and so on), the institution of monogamous marriage has been slowly crumbling for some time. Some might even say that it is well into the process of rotting away, if you define monogamy only by people's fidelity to one another. Considered the pioneer of modern sex research, Alfred Kinsey found way back in 1953 that around half of married men had cheated on their spouses, along with a quarter of married women. In 1991 Sherri Hite found that 70 per cent of married men *and* women in America cheated, although many felt this number was far too high.[168] In the past few years, statistical estimates have ranged from 25 per cent to 72 per cent of married people saying they have cheated.[169] Unmarried college students cheat too! For example, a study in the *Journal of Social and Personal Relationships* of over 500 college students in the US showed that the majority had cheated on their partners, ranging from kissing someone else (over 60 per cent of men and women) to having full-on intercourse with someone other than their partner (nearly half of men and one-third of women).[170]

The common narrative suggests that people who cheat simply lack discipline or respect for their partners, or they cheat because they are no longer in love or no longer care about their partners. While men and women cheat for a variety of reasons, most of the literature suggests that people cheat because they desire sex with someone else, even if they are still in love with their partners. Contrary to the flailing all-or-nothing narrative on fidelity, some relationship psychologists argue that it is possible to be in love with your partner, but still seek out sex from someone else. This notion shoves aside any remaining fake old news Disney movie, "Rom Com" notions of romance, where we love someone so much that we would never dream of looking at another potential mate, let alone fooling around with them. Given the damaging gender role and relationship stereotypes perpetuated by this narrative discussed earlier, perhaps this is a good thing?

Are We Rewriting the Narrative on Fidelity?

As it turns out, from an evolutionary psychology perspective, the desire for sexual variety is not only common, but inherently natural to nearly all advanced primates, including human beings! Less than 5 per cent of the 5,000 plus mammal species in existence form monogamous pair bonds, the closest to humans being the gibbon (with whom we share a few traits, socially, evolutionarily and otherwise).[171]

It remains challenging at best to find a scientific explanation for the evolution of monogamy in humans. Ever since Darwin's *On the Origin of Species*, ideas have circulated about the evolution of monogamy vis-à-vis the allocation of resources in male–female pair bonding. Because a man is inherently uncertain as to the paternity of his children due to women's hidden ovulation, he must ensure that a woman stays faithful only to him to guarantee that his resources are spent only upon his genetic descendants. And yet, are we expected to believe that this *"paternity uncertainty"* hypothesis drives modern human mating behaviour? If we are to assume, as evolutionary psychology suggests, that not only our bodies but also our behaviours are inherited from early humans, these early humans were most likely much closer to the social, sexual chimpanzees and bonobos, who are both well known for multi-male-multi-female mating.

All signs point to monogamy then, not necessarily as an evolutionary or biological adaptation, but as a cultural, social and religious one, at least for some people. Christopher Ryan and Cacilda Jethá's groundbreaking *Sex at Dawn* (2010) has put forward the hypothesis that much of our accepted narrative about human sexual prehistory could be incorrect, especially when it comes to the misconception that humans evolved to be monogamous.[172]

The most fascinating part of *Sex at Dawn* for me comes not from the comparison between human and ape mating styles, but rather from the parallels between the humans of today and the humans of the past. Indeed, the authors ask why the dominant narrative refuses to consider *"prehistoric promiscuity"* in our understanding of current human sexual behaviour, when nearly every relevant source of evidence seems to point in that direction.[173] It is widely thought (and supported by fossil records) that for hundreds of thousands of years, human beings lived in hunter gatherer societies where sharing of all resources, including mates, was not only encouraged but mandatory. According to Ryan and Jethá,

a great deal of research from primatology, anthropology, anatomy, and psychology points to the same fundamental conclusion: Human beings and our hominid ancestors have spent almost all of the past few million years or so in small, intimate bands in which most adults had several sexual relationships at any given time. This approach probably persisted until the rise of agriculture and private property no more than 10,000 years ago. In addition to voluminous scientific evidence, many explorers, missionaries and anthropologists support this view, having penned accounts rich with tales of orgiastic rituals, unflinching mate sharing, and open sexuality unencumbered by guilt or shame.[174]

If We Didn't Evolve to Be Monogamous, then What on Earth Happened!?

While the hunter gatherer societies of our past had no choice but to prioritize group identity, collective welfare and the survival of their community, in modern society we certainly do not live like this. So what happened? About 10,000 years ago, humans developed agriculture and city states began to arise, ushering in the era of possession and private property where women were owned like livestock. Suddenly, the welfare of the collective became much less important than the welfare of the individual and his direct offspring. As a man's ownership of one specific woman and her child became more important, so too did his woman's fidelity and his investment of resources only in his own biological children.

Monogamous marriage might have been an effective adaptation strategy to the changes in our society over the past 10,000 years, but it is a strategy that seems to be failing us rather dramatically given the astounding rates of cheating and divorce in modern times (indeed, nearly half of all marriages in the US now end in divorce, although the divorce rate has been falling since 2008 – but more on that in a moment). In the million+ year timeline of human evolution and existence, 10,000 years seems like a pretty small blip on the radar – a blip which has irrevocably shaped everything about who we think we are. Or has it?

Could it be that everything we think we know about human mating is wrong? Is it possible that deep within us lies that same desire for sharing and freedom that our ancestors once had? Is it likely that the current moral configuration of monogamy itself is what feels unnatural, at least to some of us?

Marking the trend of new relationship styles, millennials are choosing to get married at a far lower rate than previous generations. According to the Pew Research Center (2014), only about one-quarter of adults aged 18 to 32 in America have been married, whereas nearly half of our parents' generation were married when they were our age. Seven out of ten millennials have never married, and if we make the choice, we are waiting until an average of 27 for women and 29 for men (versus an average of 20 for women and 23 for men in 1960).[175] Because college graduates are waiting longer to get married while they focus on their careers (and on getting out of debt!), fewer overall marriages means a steady decline in divorce rates over the past ten years.[176] Preliminary statistics also indicate that Gen-Zs tend to view marriage as even *less* important than millennials do.[177]

Psychologically, socially and emotionally, divorce can be traumatizing. But are all divorces caused by cheating? Probably not. Would some of these people have divorced if they could have been non-monogamously married? Maybe. Or maybe they just were not compatible or happy together. It can be shaky ground to conflate marriage with monogamy, although that is still the traditional way of looking at pair bonding. Perhaps the very meaning of marriage is evolving to represent the transforming social and economic structures of our world, and the shift from nuclear families into something more fluid.

Consensual Non-Monogamy (CNM)

The umbrella term *consensual non-monogamy* (CNM) has evolved to describe a range of relationship styles that incorporate more than two people that all partners know about. *CNM does not mean cheating!* There are so many different types of CNM that describing them all would exceed the scope of this chapter!

However, author and CNM relationship expert Franklin Veaux recently published a map of the types of non-monogamy, which provides insight into the vast world of CNM and its many possible relationship styles.[178]

According to a 2016 analysis of nearly 10,000 census responses published in the *Journal of Sex and Marital Therapy*, 1 in 5 adults in the US reports engaging in some type of consensual non-monogamy through the course of their lives.[179] The ratios remained constant across age, education level, income, religion, region, political affiliation and race, but varied with gender and sexual orientation. Specifically, men (compared to women) and people who identify as gay, lesbian or bisexual (compared to those who identify as heterosexual) were more likely to report previous engagement in CNM. Other research has shown that 5 per cent of adults are *currently* in non-monogamous relationships, or around 10 million adults in the US.[180]

Even more intriguing is a 2016 *YouGov* poll of more than 1,000 adults in the US showing that that around half of men and one-third of women say that their ideal relationship involves some form of non-monogamy – but fewer were actually in non-monogamous relationships (around 1 in 3).[181] Non-monogamy was much more common among millennials (about half had tried it), reflecting how we are pursuing fluidity in many aspects of our love and sex lives, from our identities to our relationships.

Polyamory: Where Love and Sex Meet

The most high-profile type of CNM currently and the word on everyone's lips, *polyamory* literally means "*multiple loves*", a 1990s term that emerged as a fusion of the Greek (poly) for many, and the Latin (amor) for love. Some people still confuse polyamory with polygamy or polygyny, which are different: Polygamy is the act of having many spouses, like the sister wives of the Church of Latter-Day Saints in Utah (polygyny meaning multiple wives and polyandry meaning multiple husbands). Polyamory on the other hand is about building loving, consensual relationships with multiple people simultaneously. There are countless possible polyamorous relationship structures, and these often can feel freeform and fluid (as has been the case for me).

Consider that many people in polyamorous relationships do not necessarily place emphasis on the *relationship escalator*, which is the socially conditioned idea that people should date, fall in love, have sex, get married, buy a house together and have some kids, all in that order. In fact, whether we are polyamorous or monogamous, many of us reject the notion of following a traditional pattern that plots out the course of our lives! Instead, we are embracing more fluid ideas about who we fall in love with, and who we commit to, and why. *Ambiamory* reflects an emerging relationship trend which emphasizes people choosing relationship structures that fit the individuals involved, as well as the life situations in which they find themselves. An ambiamorous person might be happy being monogamous at some point in their lives, as well as happy being polyamorous at other times in their lives depending upon the people and situations involved. What I appreciate about this perspective is its focus on fluidity (something important to many of us!) as opposed to the rigidity of identifying with either one camp or the other. Ambiamorous people don't believe that monogamy is required for their happiness, but they also don't believe that polyamory is somehow more superior. This perspective rejects being categorized by either and instead emphasizes how relationships can fluctuate, much like our new perceptions of gender and sexuality.

In light of the growing importance of relationship fluidity, let's consider how relationship structures could evolve when people explore polyamory. Imagine a couple named Rob and Beth who have been together happily for four years. They are in their late 20s and they share an apartment together and a golden retriever named Koda. While they are committed to each other, they also have made it no secret that they find themselves sexually attracted to other people. They've even talked about what it would be like if they opened up their relationship. One day, Beth meets a guy named Max at a yoga class and they have coffee after, totally hitting it off. She's attracted to him and would love to keep hanging out, possibly seeing where this might go romantically. Beth tells Max that she already has a live-in boyfriend. She also tells Rob how she feels about Max, and because he loves her and wants to support her to explore her sexuality more deeply, they decide to open up the relationship. Beth starts hanging out with Max, and after talking to Rob about it and getting his consent first, she and Max become intimate. She even develops strong emotional feelings for him, all while remaining in her long-term relationship with Rob.

We would call this a *primary-secondary* relationship where Rob and Beth are primary partners (meaning they are in a long-term relationship together), making Beth and Max secondary partners. Now you're probably wondering, it sounds alright in theory but in practice, would this actually work? In my experience, sometimes it works and sometimes it doesn't. When it works, this is usually because of the *Coolidge Effect* (named after an old joke about President Calvin Coolidge), which is the idea from biology that sexual behaviour and response habituate over time. Beth may get so turned on by her new relationship with Max that it actually increases her satisfaction and sexual attraction to Rob as well. One of the largest ever studies on polyamorous couples found that secondary partners had sex more frequently than the primary partners did, but the primary partners experienced elevated levels of relationship investment, satisfaction and better communication.[182] In this instance, even though Beth might have been having more sex with Max than with Rob, adding Max into her life also made her feel closer to Rob and happier in her relationship with him.

If you're thinking, this is way too complicated, or, Rob's getting a raw deal, or, "I would never be happy if my partner was dating someone else!" perhaps a primary-secondary relationship would not be a good fit for you. Let's say that things fizzled out between Beth and Max. But then, at a house music show, Beth and Rob meet Rebecca, and the three of them fall in love. Rebecca is attracted to both members of the couple, but she has a closer relationship with Rob and has sex with him more frequently, even when Beth isn't around. Beth is ok with this because she loves having Rebecca around and after some deliberations, they invite Rebecca to move in with them. Sometimes all three of them have sex. Sometimes Beth and Rebecca have sex. Rebecca is not required to share her time equally between Beth and Rob (see section on unicorns later on in the chapter). We would call this a *triad*, which is the simplest form of polyamory, where three people share deep and loving relationships with one another. Another example of a relationship between three people is a *vee*, where one person serves as the pivot point between two partners. This would occur in an alternative universe where Rob is not around (sorry, Rob!) and where Beth is dating both Max and Rebecca independently. This vee could easily turn into a triad where Beth, Max and Rebecca all end up in a relationship together.

Still with me? Let's put Rob back into the picture. And let's turn back the clock and pretend that Beth and Rob never met Rebecca, and Beth never met Max at yoga. Instead, Rebecca is the one who met Max at yoga, and they have been dating for a few months. Rob, Beth, Max and Rebecca might end up in a group relationship together. Let's say that after being introduced by mutual friends and spending a lot of time together, the four of them decide to become sexually intimate, they fall in love, and they decide that they want to be together as a four-person group. This would be called a *quad* relationship, where all four members share a loving and intimate connection. Often, quads begin as two couples who merge to become a foursome. This quad might also become a *polyfidelitous* group, meaning that they agree to stay faithful to only their group.

Much like monogamy, polyfidelity reflects a closed loop where new partners are not included without everyone's consent. People choose polyfidelity for a number of reasons, such as reducing their risk of contracting STIs by exposing themselves to new partners, or to avoid unwanted pregnancies from people outside the group, or because it's taxing and time consuming enough to be in relationships with multiple people and adding more just gets confusing!

These examples (even though they are simplified) help show the fluid ways in which polyamorous relationships can emerge and evolve. There is no one-size-fits-all approach here. You are not obligated to stay in any one structure, so long as you communicate with your partner(s) about what is and isn't working for you. In recent years the concept of *relationship anarchy* (RA) has emerged, emphasizing the fluid and dynamic nature of love and sex. Some people describe RA as the "logical extreme" of polyamory, offering a less couple-centric approach, based rather upon autonomy, abundance and consent within the context of subjective and specific relationships. RA also diminishes the distinction between couples, romantic partners and "friends with benefits", emphasizing that certain relationships do not fall within prescribed roles. Some people prefer the term *relationship fluidity* over relationship anarchy, recognizing freedom of choice, inclusivity, humanity and integrity in the way we approach our different relationships.[183]

Labelling Relationship Choices

For anyone who is saying, "well, I don't want to be labelled poly or ambiamorous," or, "I'm not sure how open I want my relationship to be" and so on: We have already discussed how labels can be useful, but as sex positive people we must reject the idea that anyone's sexuality or relationship style must fit into a singular, broadly defined category. Feel free to reject any label placed upon your relationships that makes you feel uncomfortable. Or, even better, make your own label if you feel like you need one. If the category of "open" or "poly" is too much for you, but you still want to date, have sex with, or love multiple people, non-monogamous is always a good general choice to describe yourself. New permutations of non-monogamy are constantly emerging based upon people's needs and desires, so if you haven't found the label that fits you yet, wait a few years (and check Subreddit regularly!) and you will find it.

Mythbusters: Polyamory Edition

One of the most common misconceptions about polyamory (which usually comes from people who have never experienced it, fancy that!) is that the poly lifestyle operates as a sexual "free for all" where people can just do whatever they want. They don't have to ask permission; they can just go on a "fuck fest" and be totally irresponsible about it. If you ask 100 polyamorous people if this was true, at least 99 would say that this is not the case, whether in triads, quads or something else. If anything, polyamorous people tend to be excellent communicators and they work to build trust and value ethics, autonomy and consent. Obviously, the behaviours depend upon rules people set out in their relationships (which of course are always subject to change). While people on the outside might say, "Oh it must be so easy to be poly and have so much freedom!!" or "How nice, you must get to do whatever you want!" being poly is also not for the faint of heart.

Like all types of relationships, polyamory is rife with challenges and difficulties. Many of those who idealize the lifestyle imagine it being a blast but sometimes do not consider the effort involved. This is not just a weekend retreat or an easy slut utopia where anything goes. Here are some of the common misconceptions that have been brought up about being poly, for those readers who are thinking about it, or for those who, like me, are already dabbling:

Myth 1: Being Poly Requires No Sacrifices
People might think that having sex with multiple people means you get to "have it all" and never settle or sacrifice, but this could not be further from the truth. You will be giving things up, as you would in most relationships. But in poly, there might be times when one (or more) of your partners feels the need to give their attention to another,

instead of you. You might be home alone while your partner is on a date with someone else. And if you can't cope with that level of jealousy (more on that later) this might become a big huge problem.

Myth 2: Everyone Will Always Get Along
It is vital to recognize that your partners might not get along. Or you might not get along with your partners' partners. You might feel icky about them at first, but you might grow to love, or at least, respect them. I've been there, but I can tell you that using a veto to block a relationship you don't like is almost never the answer. Sometimes we agree to disagree, and sometimes we must have faith that our partner would not make such a bad decision. Everyone will not always get along and expecting anything else will cue you up for frustration down the road.

Myth 3: Poly People Are Unsatisfied
Outsiders assume that someone must be unsatisfied if they have to go outside of their relationship for love and sex. This harkens back to the normative lie we are taught about monogamy: That one person must be able to satisfy us forever, or there is something wrong with us! And yet, a survey of over 1,000 polyamorous adults in the US found that poly people were highly satisfied and felt closer and more supported by their primary partners.[184] This implies that seeking additional partners is not indicative of relationship dissatisfaction.

Myth 4: Poly People Are Gross, Creepy and Wouldn't Get Laid if They Weren't Poly
This is one of my favourite myths because there probably are creepy poly people out there, just like there probably are creepy monogamous people out there. I've seen some heater YouTube spoofs about this (Chris Fleming's *Polyamorous* cracks me up, he sings, "*It's never who you want to be*

polyamorous who is polyamorous"[185]), but isn't beauty and sexual attraction in the eye of the beholder anyway? I haven't heard many stories (if any!) about polyamorous couples trying to force themselves on unsuspecting people (but maybe I have heard these types of stories about hegemonic men, hmm?) Polyamorous people run the gamut, just like everyone else.

Coping with Jealousy

Navigating passages through jealousy could be the topic of an entire book when it comes to polyamory, and in my experience, it is people's most frequent concern when opening up their relationships. Jealousy is not an emotion or skill we are taught to manage or learn: If anything, because of our conditioned fears about acceptance, jealousy is a part of life, and it is even encouraged as a method to stoke competition in some arenas.

Consider the idea of *compersion*, defined as the opposite of jealousy, or, a feeling of joy at your partner's joy of sex and love with other people.[186] When you feel that deeply uncomfortable twinge of jealousy, first remember that it is a completely natural feeling. Don't beat yourself up. Instead, try to think about the underlying psychology of what is really bothering you: Are you afraid your partner is going to leave you for someone else, or that they are having more fun with someone else? Are you angry because you are missing out? Do you have to be number one, and you think you might be unseated? Do you have deep wounds of abandonment that are being triggered? Do you want to scream, punch someone or smash up your house? Or do you just feel gross inside and can't quite put your finger on it? When you start to feel the unpleasantness creep in, take some deep breaths, sit with yourself, connect to your emotions, and write in your journal (if you keep one) about exactly how you feel.

If we can address the causes of our jealousies and begin to target the sources of the discomfort, then the next step to compersion involves learning to live with your jealousy, as opposed to pretending it does not exist as it bubbles and festers deep below the surface. Denying your emotions (whether it's jealousy or something else), bottling them up or projecting them upon your partner(s), are not the types of healthy emotional coping strategies that will enable you to bring more compersion into your life.

Because open relationships can feel so experiential and subjective, some people might not even notice the triggers of jealousy until they are right smack in the middle of a sexual or romantic situation unfolding between their partner and someone else. Fitness and lifestyle guru Aubrey Marcus (who is polyamorous, by the way!) told me in an interview *to follow the resistance!* In other words, when we have these terrible, unpleasant, uncomfortable feelings about something, there is probably a lot we can learn about ourselves by pursuing the source of the feelings and making some self-discoveries or resolutions about these feelings.

Remember that you do not have control over who people fall in love with (even you, ha!). So much jealousy in all types of relationships comes from the fear of losing someone: But remember, they were never really "yours" to begin with! Embracing this belief is what has helped me to love without fear, and even become extremely turned on by compersion. If my partner(s) are being pleasured by someone in a way that makes them happy, I can't really ask for anything more. Take note that this process of letting go of control over other people's happiness requires real emotional work but can improve many areas of your life. So be patient and kind to yourself. Ride out the storm when it happens and keep trying. You can get there.

Unicorns (Mythical Creatures)

A *unicorn* is best defined as a "hot bi babe" (HBB) or as a "hypothetical woman who is willing to be involved with members of an existing couple, to have no relationships other than with the members of that couple, to not be sexually involved with one member of the couple unless the other member of the couple is also there, and who usually moves in with the couple."[187]

Usually when couples first open up their relationships, a plethora of fears and insecurities can erupt over what happens if one person finds another partner first, while the other has to wait around twiddling their thumbs (or holding their proverbial dicks in proverbial hands) while their lover is out on sexy dates and getting laid. Generally, if you are in a primary-secondary relationship then it would be strange if both people found outside partners at exactly the same time. (Spoiler alert: In a heterosexual couple it is usually the female who finds an outside partner first, like our example with Rob and Beth.)

One of the common ways that couples try to overcome their natural fears and insecurities about sharing their partners is to present themselves as a "unit" or a package deal, where they dip their joint fishing lines in the poly waters by baiting a hook for a single, bisexual woman who they can both date ... together. For some men, introducing another penis to the situation can be uncomfortable at first (thanks in part to the patriarchal notion of men "owning" their women). In fact, multiple people have poly arrangements that institute a "*one penis policy*" where a man may have sex with multiple female partners but the woman is forbidden to become intimate with any other man (and yet, a female who has a group of male partners where no other vaginas are allowed seems extremely rare. Funny huh?) Bringing in another woman without the alleged threat of another man sounds like it could offer a safe, controlled way to open up a relationship.

But if this is your ideal form of polyamory, you're probably out of luck. Many couples out there continue to search for their special unicorn at various poly play parties or on group dating websites and become frustrated when they can't find one. Now I'm not saying that unicorns don't exist, but they are mythically rare indeed. Many women in poly circles will say *no* to the arrangement because the whole idea emphasizes couple privilege. How? The primary couple sets all the terms and rules, and the unicorn is forced to obey them or leave. Demanding equal love and equal sex time from a partner so that one or both people in the primary relationship avoid feeling jealousy or insecurity is not what being poly is all about.

With all this talk about unicorns in male–female couples where only the woman is bisexual ... We have to wonder, are there gay and lesbian couples out there who are also looking for unicorns? Sure. The dream of having a third partner who safely gives equal love and sex to both members of a couple extends beyond all genders and sexual orientations. When it comes to wanting a controlled, safe poly experience, it is natural for people to think that this would be an acceptable option. Don't feel bad if this was the ideal form of poly you were looking for, just manage your expectations. And remember, we cannot control who people love, or how they love, or make them love in the exact way that we want! Once you open up to being poly, you must let go of control and go with the flow.

The New Relationship Energy and Polyamory

Remember what you read in the last chapter about the New Relationship Energy (NRE)? Well, the NRE can pose a whole host of intricate problems for non-monogamous people (but it is not necessarily the death knell of these relationships!). If you're already attached, and you're feeling this amazing, giddy, lovey energy for someone else, you might end up making bad decisions, neglecting your other relationship(s), or just not being in the mood to romp anymore with your other partner when you get home. Some poly people even describe themselves (or others) like addicts, or NRE junkies, jumping from new relationship to new relationship to help prolong that lascivious glow. This can be damaging to both themselves and their partner's psyches, when we treat people like sparklers to be used and then discarded when the flame runs out.

If you're going to fall in love with multiple people at once, it is important to manage your expectations about the NRE/

honeymoon period, whether it is you who gets the glow up, or your partner. When it comes to the NRE, please keep some considerations in mind. Ignoring your other partner in favour of your shiny new toy is not the best way to go. Yes, enjoy the new energy while it lasts, but not at the expense of your other partners. They need to know they are still valued and respected even when you don't have time for them because you're wrapped up in the exciting vibes with someone else. Remember, even though you might be feeling this energy, your partner might find themselves in the same space in the future. Good communication and trust are the key for navigating this energy. Who knows what tomorrow could bring?

Redefining the Relationships of the Future

From "group Tinder" to Couples Seeking Singles/Couples on OKCupid, non-monogamy is not going anywhere, particularly amongst millennials and Gen-Z. With the greatest ever number of sexually active adult humans reporting their involvement in and desire for CNM, we can only expect that the culture and community surrounding non-monogamy will continue to grow and evolve. While it is unclear what the future holds for new types of fluid relationships, the biggest part of the excitement here is the novelty, and the ability to choose your own adventures. Just remember that non-monogamy is not better, more evolved, smarter or more spiritual than monogamy: Being sex positive means that each of us has the right to choose the relationship structure that best works for us! If you're into exploring this, focus on your intentions. Be a good communicator. The future of sex positive relationships is wide open and filled with magical possibilities, as well as potential fuck buddies, lovers, partners and friends. But we need to address one of the biggest limitations to our new relationships and how to overcome it: The ways in which we communicate almost exclusively via technology.

CHAPTER 9
REWRITING THE RELATIONSHIP SCRIPT

It is undeniable that the entire millennial dating landscape has shifted drastically in the past two decades or so, from something that existed entirely IRL (in real life) to something that is now constructed, negotiated and agreed upon via social media and online dating. The sheer power and irresistibility of social media means that we often allow ourselves to expand into situations that we would never even consider IRL, which can lead to a variety of outcomes, ranging from beneficial to harmful, especially when it comes to sex and relationships!

Take the way that technology has infiltrated the bedroom. We already know that we might be having slightly less sexual intercourse than previous generations when they were our age, but my goodness, we are certainly spending way more time sexting, watching porn and snapping dick pics. It's pretty clear that as the options we have to connect with one another have expanded, so too have we begun to evolve in how we meet our sexual needs, and how we communicate about these needs. How do we meet a potential new partner? We download a dating app. And how do we demonstrate our worth on said dating app? Through a couple of our best pictures and a short bio that nobody really reads.

Direct social media marketing has taken over not only the way that products are sold in this tech savvy brave new world, but the way that human relationships are built and maintained. We have transitioned rapidly into a space where we create, tailor and distribute the images we disseminate on social media with the intention of generating sales: Not product sales per se, but the *sale of our identities* in exchange for likes, positive feedback and maybe a booty pic or a real-life date if we're lucky. We are selling ourselves to potential intimate partners, friends and fuck buddies and we are doing it knowingly, through online dating apps like Tinder and Bumble, or with our snaps or posts on the Gram. The meteoric rise of the "influencer" mindset has made us (falsely?) believe that you too can become a rich, famous celebrity just by scripting your identity into a brand and posting really lit memes, makeup tutorials, fitness videos, video game explanations or whatever people are into at the moment. Have we relinquished our real-life autonomy in favour of socially constructed artificial identities designed to literally sell ourselves to the public for instant gratification? It sure seems that way. But perhaps the real questions we need to be asking are: How is this process affecting our wellbeing? Are we feeling better or worse about ourselves and our ability to relate with others? Can we still build meaningful relationships with one another? And how do we conceptualize and understand these relationships?

A Whole New Script

To answer that question, our first stop on this whirlwind tour of online dating life begins with the brand spanking new language that we have scripted seemingly overnight to describe our new realities. We've created a whole new vernacular to describe everything about dating, while making sure to distinguish all of our connections from actually ever resembling dating! As a generation we seem to feel inherently distrustful of getting too close to people, and our new dating language seems to reflect it in its entirety.

Have you ever noticed how the term "talking" seems to have altogether replaced the word "dating"? "I've been talking to a guy" can mean anything from literally chatting online to full-on hooking up, but basically, we're mostly all about keeping it casual. Does anyone nowadays want to admit they are actually dating anyone, let alone asserting themselves in a full-on relationship? It makes me laugh when I think about my parents teasing me in middle school me about "going steady" with a boy. Does anyone want commitment anymore? The jury is still out on that one, but if you think about the new slang, the answer seems pretty clear.

Dick Moves

A lot of the new vernacular invokes the increasingly crappy ways that people stop "talking" – notice I didn't say "break up"! One of the benefits to being so noncommittal every step of the way is that there isn't the same need to explicitly *end* a relationship. Thanks to technology, people can be completely avoidant in the ways that they break a connection and totally get away with it! Take a term most people are familiar with in our modern slang, *ghosting*. This is basically when you're "talking" with someone and they never respond or hit you back up. Like a freaking ghost, they are gone into the ether never to be seen again. But did you know that it doesn't just end with ghosting? No, there are multitudinous deviations of avoidant dating language and behaviour emerging this year, which I call "dick moves" (no insult to the male genitalia of course, females can be equally responsible for these), including:

- *Zombieing*: When someone ghosts you, but then suddenly pops up in your DMs after an extended period of no contact. Here they are, back from the dead like a zombie! They might say, "*Hey what's up, sorry I haven't been in touch,*" only to then go back into the ground and disappear once more until the next zombie-pocalypse.

- *Curving*: Curving came onto the scene a few months ago as the "new way to reject someone", which might actually be worse than ghosting itself. The premise here is that someone ghosts you when you try to make plans, but then responds to your offer to hang out several days after you sent it, usually with an excuse like "*love to see you, just been super busy.*" So, you think, Yay! This person isn't ghosting me, and you try to make plans again. Of course, the same thing happens again, and you might receive another text in two weeks asking to make plans again, but then they flake or don't reply. Over and over. The goal? Eventually you will just give and realize they were never interested. Why would someone do this instead of just saying, "*hey, I'm not that interested*"? I'm not totally sure, because it seems like a giant jerk-off session and not in a good way. They probably weren't "*too busy*" to reply when you consider how frequently people are on their phones. More likely, this was a power trip on their part. They probably want the ego boost of rejecting you, over and over. And perhaps they are also trying to keep their options open, serially curving multiple people at once?

- *Orbiting*: Similar to curving, this is when someone ghosts you, but continues to interact with your social media, liking or commenting on your posts. Hence, they are "orbiting" around you, but you never actually connect. Again, are they doing this to remind you that they are out there, still rejecting you? Maybe. This is also called *haunting*, when a ghost pops up of nowhere to spook you out on social media.

- *Phubbing*: This happens when you're hanging out with someone IRL and they are giving far more attention to their phone than you. If you've been on the receiving end of this, you already know how invalidating it can feel. Why do we do this even when we're in the presence of real people who we actually like? Are we just addicted to the rush of dopamine we get from people liking our posts on social media? Or are we trying to check people and show them they are just not that special?

- *Stashing*: This refers to hiding your partner(s) or keeping your partner secret from your friends, co-workers or families. Sure, there are a variety of reasons for doing this, like if you're just a "private person", or if you're already married, or maybe your friends or family don't know yet that you're gay/bi and you want to stay in the closet. This isn't anything new, but the fact that we now have an accepted word for it suggests it might be more common than ever.

- *Cushioning*: The best way to describe this is akin to someone who thinks they can play all sides or beat the odds to make sure they are never alone. Really stemming from an insecure attachment mental state, a person who is cushioning is purposely flirting with multiple people online or via text, even if they might currently be in a committed relationship. This way, they will have an actual cushion to fall upon, in case the current relationship doesn't work out.

- *Benching*: Along the same line of semi-twisted insecure thinking, benching involves maintaining contact with a person you know you're not that into, just in case they might one day rise to their hidden potential. Essentially, you're benching someone when you know it isn't going to work, but you don't want to completely cut them off or ghost them just in case they might suddenly become cool, or useful in some way. If someone is benching you, they aren't ghosting you, but they are probably putting in the least amount of effort necessary to keep you feeling special and around.

Some of the new relationship slang has less to do with one person being let down, and more to do with how technology is changing our relationships:

- *Textlationship*: Pretty self-explanatory, this is a relationship that occurs almost entirely via text message or DM. Maybe you've met once or twice in person, but you text daily. Maybe you met on a dating app and still haven't connected IRL but you're chatting all day on Messenger. Given that some people choose to find themselves in relationships with entirely AI or virtual partners, at least there's another person on the other end of the phone (we hope!).

- *Instagranding*: Something that we see all too often, instagranding refers to posting on social media with hopes of attracting a certain someone's attention. This can mean posting sexy selfies hoping that special guy will see them or sharing IG live stories of being at a cool show hoping it will raise your social capital with the girl you like. According to a 2019 *Plenty of Fish* survey, more than two-thirds of 25-year-old online daters admit tailoring the posts on the social media to attract a potential mate.[188] This also includes one of my least favourite online behaviours, *vaguebooking* needy posts, where someone posts something like, "*I'm so bored and lonely, who wants to take me out?*" only to get lots of offers but turning them all down because the post was clearly meant for someone specific or meant to drum up self-esteem through attention with no actual intention of following through.

Although most of our dating slang might make it seem like our dating worlds are horribly narcissistic, avoidant and fake, it's not always that bad. Some of the new dating language actually evokes feelings of love and connectedness, even if it's only temporary:

- *Breezing*: This refers to being open minded and not wanting to play games, something you would express as you're starting a new relationship, wanting it to keep it "breezy". Yes, our dating world is so twisted that we actually need a phrase for people who are seeking to openly express their feelings! Being ready to breeze someone means you want to just be able to hang out, talk, and get it on without worrying about what it means in the future. This is still noncommittal AF but at least we are being upfront about it!

- *Penguins*: Animal fans out there know that penguins mate for life in monogamous pair bonds, so when you've found that person that you really want to be with long term, they are your penguin, and the two of you are "penguining".

- *Cuffing season*: Ah, save the best for last. Cuffing season typically occurs in the fall/winter months, when many people who were out playing the field or avoiding commitment decide that when the holidays come into play, they don't want to be left alone out in the cold. For winter season then, some people seek to get "cuffed" or tied down into a relationship. Cuffing season is preceded by *drafting season*, when people take stock of their potential mates and decide which one would be the best to be cuffed to for the winter. And after cuffing season ends? Well of course we have *uncuffing season,* where the weather warms up, the genitals thaw out, and we want to go hit all the parties and the bars and be single again. So yes, in a nutshell, cuffing season is the time of year when single people shack up, basically using each other to avoid feeling alone, only to usually end it so they can get out there and have fun in the summer.

To put it bluntly, social media may have given us too much power to act like douchebags by offering us new ways to magnify our avoidant and narcissistic behaviours. If you've ever been ever ghosted or curved, you know it hurts. But without any real accountability on social media, maybe it makes sense that we are becoming less willing to actually commit to each other? This is beginning to feel like a vicious cycle that we can only break by deciding that we are going to treat people with the same amount of respect and attention that we feel we deserve. If we truly want to live more sex positive lives, we owe it to ourselves, our friends and our partners to use social media conversations more responsibly. After all, none of these behaviours are new, it's just that social media enables us to engage in them much more frequently. Maybe to figure out how to repair our communications, we also need to understand how online communication has rewired our brains to constantly seek reward or punishment for certain words and actions.

Online Communication: Harmful Addiction or Useful Tool?

To understand how social media and online dating have drastically altered the way in which we communicate and build relationships, let us consider the nature of the Internet itself. As mentioned earlier, many social media users are consciously or subconsciously creating and selling branded versions of themselves for attention, affection and self-esteem. We have been trained and conditioned to believe that positive attention on social media means we are good, important people, whereas negative attention or no attention means that nobody cares about us.

According to the *uses and gratifications* approach in sociology, the extent to which our use of media gives us personal gratification is the extent to which we will continue to utilize it. And we know that when people log into Instagram, seeing those love hearts and comments pop up in bright red actually triggers a dopamine response (similar to cocaine, alcohol and cannabis) that gives us a feeling of reward. And when we don't have that reward? A 2017 study published in *PLOS One* found that frequent Internet users experienced significant physiological changes, including increased heart rate and blood pressure, as well as anxiety, when their internet usage was terminated.[189] These physiological changes in many ways mirrored those of a drug addict going into withdrawal. Similarly, a 2011 study of 1,000 college students across ten countries found that 4 out of 5 respondents reported "significant mental and physical distress, panic, confusion and extreme isolation" when they were asked to unplug from technology for an "entire" day. To describe their experiences of turning off social media, they used analogies like "going cold turkey" and "itching like a crackhead", and even reported physical symptoms like panic attacks and heart palpitations.[190]

Scientists at Imperial College London have speculated that as many as 10 per cent of internet users are "addicted" meaning that they cannot control their compulsive internet usage, although tracking is hard because the concept of an "internet use disorder" is still quite new in psychology. The term "Smartphone Syndrome" has even emerged to describe the mental health crisis of being too connected and spending too much time on our phones (many of us spend more than six hours per day in front of a screen).[191] According to a 2015 report from the Pew Research Center, 94 per cent of teens in the US spend time with friends on social media, with 1 in 3 saying that they spend time with friends on social media every day. More than 8 out of 10 of these teen social media users agreed that social media allows people to show a different side of their personality, with nearly that many saying that people are less authentic on social media than they are in real life.[192]

While we know that our interactions might be somewhat fake, we are still using social media to connect with our friends and we still take it pretty damn seriously. Is this inherently problematic? Not necessarily. It becomes problematic when we fail to take into account the ways in which *online disinhibition* shapes all forms of social media communication and dialogue. Coined by psychologist Dr John Suler, online disinhibition shows how our virtual communication differs from real-life communication in certain critical ways, including dissociative anonymity, invisibility and asynchronicity:

- *Dissociative anonymity*: It is easy to hide and remain anonymous in social media, indeed, many users do not use their real names or photos, and users who post comments on YouTube, Reddit and such are also under no obligation to use their real names. This anonymity is dissociative because when posting comments or interacting online, users often do not have to take personal responsibility for their comments. This can lead to more extreme and intense conversations than people would be willing to engage in when face to face, opening up a whole potential world of trolling, harassment and triggering every time we log on.

- *Invisibility*: It is possible to remain completely invisible in certain social media environments. Whether you are viewing someone's profile or page, watching videos or reading the comments on a thread, you don't have to worry about how you look, how you sound or how people perceive your body language. Often there is a level of passive participation, when you can be viewing someone's page, pictures or comments … and this person does not even know that you exist! Suddenly, we can all be creepers or get creeped on, often without even realizing it.
- *Asynchronicity*: Unlike in real life, social media interactions do not necessarily happen in real time. Often, there can be a delay of hours or days in between comments, giving people plenty of time to come up with witty responses, or worse, leave you hanging. People can put ideas or hurtful comments out there in a type of "emotional hit and run" where they can just make these remarks, and then run away and ignore your response. This definitely wouldn't fly in real life, where we have to be sharp and tuned in at all times, and where our words and actions have actual palpable consequences.[193]

The outcome? Because of online disinhibition, we are conditioning ourselves to communication styles that leave us more open to hurt, conflict and trolling, without the human experiences of validation and compassionate understanding to balance us out. People can creep, they can say nasty things, and they have unbridled access to our lives like never before. With this level of vulnerability comes a resistance to truly get close to anyone, which possibly explains why our dating slang reflects many ideas about avoidant half-assed commitment. But what happens when we actually are trying to make a connection with someone on online dating? Does this vulnerability still get the best of us?

Online Dating and Self Esteem: The Harsh Truth

On the surface, online dating sounds like the best idea ever. Find love without leaving your house! Scroll in your PJs with a glass of wine on the couch and you can find a match of your dreams! Or find love while you're playing *Call of Duty* and drinking a six pack. The catch? On Tinder, we know that if you swipe right (meaning you like someone you see), they have to swipe right on you too in order for you to match. Usually, people make these matches arbitrarily based upon a few photos and a short bio that nobody really reads, or they just do it out of boredom or because they are seeking attention. On some platforms, like Bumble, a man can only message a woman if they both match and she messages him first. And on other platforms, like Grindr and Scruff (for gay men), all you have to do is log on to experience a veritable dickpic-pocalypse! Last week, as I was hanging out with a friend of mine, he showed me no fewer than 40 unsolicited dick pics sent to him on Grindr after being on the app for less than five minutes. Wowzah.

Now whether this sounds like an awesome way to meet people or a heinous waste of time to you, this hasn't stopped online dating from becoming the new norm of how many of us look to find love, fuck buddies or just to get attention and ego boosts. Consider some staggering statistics: In 2019, Tinder claims to have generated 1.6 billion swipes per day worldwide, leading to 26 million daily matches, and over 1 million dates per week. Nearly two-thirds of their active daily users are men.[194] The vast majority (nearly 8 out of 10!) of all Tinder users are millennials aged 18 to 36. The number one reason that millennials use Tinder according to a 2017 survey of 3,500 US college students? Entertainment, followed by casual dating and ego boosts.[195]

In this survey, 13 per cent of college students on Tinder admitted that they did it for the ego boost (and this was similar across other sites Bumble and OkCupid). If we think about how absolutely massive online dating has become, with billions of swipes and millions of matches per day, we should consider how the majority of college students could be using it for reasons described as somewhat narcissistic or just plain disingenuous. Since over half of college-aged users admitted that they are using Tinder just for entertainment and ego boosts, should we be concerned that the people who are actually looking for love or casual relationships might be putting themselves into a vulnerable position that could damage their self-esteem should they take a genuine interest in someone? Or should we all know better, that online dating apps like Tinder are really more about avoiding boredom and making ourselves feel special?

Whether we do know better or not, startling research has emerged showing how using Tinder can actually damage people's self-esteem. A 2017 study published in the journal *Body Image* of nearly 1,300 college aged students in the US showed that regardless of gender, Tinder users scored significantly lower on measures of self-worth than non-Tinder users, including indicators like body satisfaction, self-esteem, feelings of body shame, internalization of cultural beauty standards, comparisons to others and self-objectification.[196] Even more surprising? Male Tinder users had the lowest self-esteem, even lower than female Tinder users. Even for men with high self-esteem, the researchers noted that "the current Tinder system does not work in their favour."[197]

What is going on here? One might expect women's self-esteem to be most adversely affected by online dating, considering women's social conditioning and acceptance of societal beauty standards. And yet, Tinder use affects men even more adversely than women. How? One of the problems is how there are way more men on Tinder than women, meaning that men are more likely to get rejected based upon supply and demand alone. This also means that some (but not all) of the women on Tinder are getting more attention than they do IRL, thanks to the extreme gender imbalance on the app. Furthermore, the researchers explained that men swipe right much more frequently than women do, which means that they are subjected to a much higher incidence of rejection. And if you've ever been rejected online, you know that *rejection is rejection*! In person or online, it can hurt. It can hurt so bad that one 2011 study actually showed how being socially rejected triggers the same part of the brain as physical pain.[198] Social rejection literally shares the same somatosensory representation as being physically hurt, meaning it is harder than we had previously thought for us to cognitively tell the difference between a broken heart or a bruised ego and a punch in the face or a broken bone. So why is Tinder hurting men so badly? Because instead of being rejected two or three times in one night by a few women in the club, men on Tinder might get rejected 20 times in one hour if they don't match with anyone they swiped on. Ouch.

Of course, it is also possible that people with low self-esteem naturally gravitate to online dating, creating a self-fulfilling prophecy of rejection that reinforces their unworthiness. I'd like to see a comparison between the self-esteem of gay men who use Grindr and those who do not, just to find out if it is the gender imbalance creating this Tinder problem, as in, heterosexual women might be doing this to boost their confidence at the expense of heterosexual men. Women absolutely have the upper hand when it comes to online dating because they are outnumbered on most apps by at a ratio of at least 2:1. Indeed, a 2018 Norwegian study of 641 college students age 19–29 showed that while men's main motivation to use dating apps was for sex, women's was more for the attention, even when they had no intention of actually ever dating anyone.[199] This also makes me wonder if female-centric dating apps like Bumble create an even sharper drop in men's self-esteem.

One of the other jarring issues pointing to the damaging effects of online dating is the high frequency of creeping, harassment and stalking that some users experience. Due to the features of online disassociation mentioned earlier, putting yourself out there on dating apps can make you a target of attentions you'd rather not receive. In that same 2017 survey of 3,500 US college students, 1 in 3 females, 1 in 6 males and over half of gender fluid people reported being harassed across online dating apps (reflecting over one-quarter of all dating app users). The highest frequency of harassment? Grindr, where more than half of all users said that they had been harassed, probably due to the app's largely unrestricted messaging features. On Grindr, you don't have to match with a guy on there for him to send you lots and lots of unsolicited dick pics (hence the dickpic-pocalypse I mentioned earlier). But is anyone really safe from harassment on online dating apps? With cyberstalking at an all-time high (approximately 1 million women and 370,000 men reporting online stalking and harassment each year), it is hardly surprising how online dating apps that facilitate one-on-one direct non-anonymous messaging would open the door for harassment. It also makes me wonder whether dating-app users' self-esteem was lower in the previous study because they were being victimized or harassed?

As a psychologist who cares about mental health, it is hard for me to turn away from the findings that online dating apps might actually have a toxic impact upon wellbeing and self-worth. I'm not saying you should delete the apps entirely if you enjoy using them, but please consider how you are putting yourself out there to be at the worst rejected, used and/or stalked, whereas at best you might get a date with someone you actually like. Maybe you haven't tried lately, but you absolutely have what it takes to meet someone IRL! These apps just serve to reinforce the emergence of the avoidant, narcissistic model of communication and dating, especially when we go out of our way to try to connect and then our attempts are invalidated or rejected. Even though the communication is virtual, the pain is still real. Ask yourself, do I really deserve to put myself through this? And if you are reading this and feeling like, "Wow, maybe this is affecting my self-esteem," delete the apps for a couple of weeks and see if you feel better. If you were only on there for entertainment or ego boost anyway, perhaps there are other, more constructive ways to achieve this?

The Psychology of Social Media and Sexual Relationships

As we move into the future, our love lives, friendships and general relationships will become increasingly intertwined with forms of technological expression that can bring us closer together while also having the potential to cause immense amounts of unintentional harm.

Are you one of the older millennials like me who was in high school in the 1990s? If you examine the ways that high school students use social media and technology today, you might feel forever grateful that there was no Facebook, no Twitter, no Instagram, no Snapchat, not even Myspace really, when we were in high school. To this day, there exists no documented accessible public record of the things I did in high school, and thankfully word of mouth has a way of fading away after 20+ years!

Sure, I was slut shamed, but if I had been slut shamed all over the internet today, it might be hanging over me like a cloud I could never delete, erase or escape from. The biggest difference growing up today versus 20 years ago lies in the way that today our experiences are publicly documented and recorded for the consumption of those in our peer groups, and for the world more broadly. Instead of having a personal diary that nobody but you can read (or your mom, if she snoops), today everything you do is recorded in the public diary we call social media where people can comment, save your images or videos and (gasp!) take screenshots.

How can we begin to understand the psychology of these changes in the way people understand and access their multiple in-person and online identities? We know that most of us rely upon social media to build and maintain our friendships, and that many do so on a daily (even hourly!) basis. Aside from transitional generations like mine (the "Xennials," born from 1977 to 1983) who only had access to crappy dial up and email in high school, every generation after has grown up having to juggle the arduous task of maintaining an in-person identity along with an online, social media persona or presence. The kicker? According to the Pew Research Center, just under half of all teens feel significant pressure to post popular or flattering content associated with their social media identity. Balancing these multiple identities can be an arduous, confusing and sometimes draining task.[200]

While most of us love social media, and cannot imagine our lives without it (indeed, various surveys have suggested that many of us may have panic attacks when forced to go without social media for only one day), I can't help but wonder if the current evolution of our technology is creating a verifiable paradise lost, a degradation of innocence where one mistake can ruin your life, and where your entire existence can be scrutinized, analysed, trolled, exalted, or crushed with a few simple key strokes. Aren't we feeling the dissonance of absolute freedom paired with the extreme pressure of this way of life? Could this be part of the reason why CDC recently found that teen suicide rates are currently at an all-time high?[201]

We know that technology challenges our inhibitory control, with smartphones and social media acting like a stimulating drug offering immediate, consistent reinforcement and gratification. (Porn addiction might be questionable but social media addiction seems real, although, is it an addiction if everyone is doing it?) Pair this with the fact that most of us are sexually active or at least seeking to experiment with our sexualities. Can you remember being an adolescent and how exciting or alluring sex was as your hormones worked on overdrive and your body began to develop? The combination of a horny teen with media that offers instant access to share graphic content with potential partners feels like a type of kryptonite that would be as alluring as it can be destructive. Add into the mix the fact that for most of us today, online, text or email communication is our preferred source of interaction: We now prefer to make and keep friends online rather than in person.[202]

Thriving in Our New Relationships

So, what does the future look like for those of us who like to use social media as the main source to pursue love, relationships and/ or sexual goals? It is highly unlikely that social media is going away anytime soon; If anything, in the future it will become more ingrained in our daily routines and more frequently utilized to engage with potential partners. This in and of itself is not a bad thing, but it can become toxic when we find ourselves slipping into the avoidant, narcissistic patterns that have been so clearly reinforced by our new language and approach to dating. Still, each of us has a choice to become part of the problem or part of the solution, by demanding respect for ourselves and offering it to others. I hate to imagine a future where we are unable to communicate in person, where the "textlationship" becomes the norm and where we can't meet people outside of dating apps or social media, but perhaps there is hope and a way of avoiding this potential fate!

Based upon all of my research, interviews and lifetime spent as a human being who has loved, lost and interacted in this brave new social environment, I wholeheartedly believe that we can overcome the confusion and isolation implied by our new styles of connecting to build empowered, happy, sex positive relationships. Even though our new modes of communication might seem overly negative and avoidant, let us not forget that the way we interact now serves as an adaptation to the media that we have become accustomed to using. If the technosexual revolution has taught us anything, it should be that we still love the feeling of connection, even if we are going through less conventional channels to get there. The need to feel loved, heard and accepted is never going away, we are just shifting in the way that we seek it out, experience it, and offer it to others. Psychological research has consistently shown that social isolation is one of the largest predictors of sickness and death, equivalent in some studies to the negative health consequences of smoking 15 cigarettes a day.[203] In other words, we will always need human connection to survive and to thrive. And even in the face of the changing attitudes about love and sex, we can still forge meaningful connections! How do we move forward here, empowering ourselves to better cope with the shifting nature of human relationships? These are the five best tips I can offer you:

Tip 1: Truly Know What You Want
Just like the deep self-work we covered in chapter 6, we must get into alignment with ourselves and our needs before we decide to enter into a relationship with another person. Remember those pesky learned behaviour patterns and programmed self-limiting beliefs? We must learn to identify those so we can see clearly if the potential relationship or partner we are seeking offers us a way to grow past those patterns or a path to remaining stuck in them. In light of all of the relationship styles discussed in this book, are you finding yourself closer to deciding what you truly want? Do you want … a soul mate? A polyamorous triad? A karmic relationship? The next Beyoncé–Jay Z power couple match-up? A sex doll or virtual partner? Someone for cuffing season? Or do you just want to be single or want something else entirely?

If you don't know what you want, then you may not be ready to get into a relationship right now. If you're in a relationship, you might want to take it slow and reflect on your feelings so you can articulate more clearly what you want. Sometimes it can help to visualize not the ideal partner themselves, but the way you would *feel* in the relationship that you seek. Would you feel sexy and desired? Or supported? Or maybe you would feel challenged to grow? Would you feel like all or your needs are being met? Or would you feel deeply independent? Asking yourself these types of questions and being genuine in your responses can help you know more deeply exactly what you want, and help you chart the best way to get there.

Tip 2: Get Out There and Find Your Tribe
Psychologically, we need a sense of community to thrive. So, find your tribe of like-minded people who share similar interests! It might feel like we have lost access to our communities in the virtual age, but we haven't. Everyone is still out there, and it is pretty easy to find them. They are out there doing real things in the real world, and most of these activities will lead you to building genuine human connections rather than the ones filtered by the medium of the Internet. As they say, your vibe will find your tribe. You have to put the effort in, not just online but also IRL! Spending time in social environments surrounded by like-minded people will open you up to a better understanding of what you want in relationships and expose you to the types of people who can offer it to you. No excuses here because everyone can do this, and meeting people IRL means more than just getting drunk at bars.

If you're into music, then going to artist showcases and small venue music events is a great way to meet people, as is volunteering to work at festivals. If you're into art, check out an art walk or a gallery or museum opening. If you're into movement arts, join a circus group or a hooping squad, or a burlesque dancing troop. If you're into sports, there are many fun co-ed volleyball and kick-ball teams out there. A friend of mine who recently had a tough breakup just joined an axe-throwing league, and she's obsessed (and has been on several dates with people she met in the league, no less). If you want to experiment sexually, there are tons of groups out there offering bondage and Shibari rope classes, as well as swingers' groups and other open or non-monogamous community groups. You'd be amazed at who you might meet if you just take the first step to get out there.

What about people who believe that their tribe only exists online, like gamers? I'll never forget an episode of the new *Queer Eye* where a young gamer didn't really have any human connections in real life. The Fab 5 brought him to a meet-up of people in his town who liked gaming and anime! Suddenly he made friends right there in person, even though their interests were virtual. Although many of us believe that we can benefit from online communication, we are also not robots. (Not yet, anyway!) We are flesh and blood humans and in order to be fulfilled, we need to build bridges and connections with other real-life humans who share our interests, where we can read each other's body language, stare into each other's eyes, and maybe even fall in love.

Tip 3: Be Crystal Clear

Don Miguel Ruiz spoke in *The Four Agreements* about being "*impeccable*" with your word and this remains crucial to building and maintaining sex positive relationships. We must be honest about our feelings, and we must mean what we say and say what we mean. For example, rise above all of the avoidant nonsense that people might be doing on Tinder. If you like someone, be direct. Don't play games. Just tell them how you feel or ask them out. If you don't like someone or don't want to keep "talking", just tell them the truth! Don't ghost them. Honesty will get you everywhere, and it will lighten the burden that you are carrying when you feel like you can't express yourself. If you want to be in an open relationship, then tell your partner the truth (instead of going behind their back and doing it anyway). If you want to try flogging, pegging or anything sexual, communicate it. If we cannot be honest, we will never be happy in our relationships. If we want to be heard, we must give people the chance to actually hear us, which means we have to stop beating around the bush and just be direct about what we want. We do ourselves and our partners a disservice by not being honest. We have to give them the chance to accept us as we seek to accept ourselves.

Being clear applies not only to your communication with others, but also to your inner dialogue with yourself. You might know what you want, but do you know how you are going to get there? Make a clear plan that will lead you to your relationship goals. Maybe this involves practising the self-love exercises from chapter 6 once per week. Or perhaps your plan entails learning your partner's love language, or maybe it just means building the type of sex positive relationship that really resonates with you. Cut out all of the noise and the programming and just get clear with yourself about how the decisions you make are going to plot the course of your life and the relationships in it.

Tip 4: Stop Apologizing!
We can thank the socialization of our sexual identities for the ways in which we are always apologizing for being ourselves. If you really want sex positive relationships in your life, then you must stop apologizing for who you are and *own your truth*, even when it scares you a little bit. Standing in your truth is the single most powerful weapon you have against unhappiness, loneliness and judgement. This probably sounds counterintuitive because often when we stand up for ourselves or we tell the truth without apologizing, we alienate people and piss them off. But maybe we are just pissing off the people that we don't need in our lives. The right people will embrace you as you own your power and stop apologizing for who you are, not only in terms of your sexuality but in terms of all areas of your identity.

I'll never forget being at a workshop many years ago in Joshua Tree where the speaker, a friend of mine named Dr Dream, was talking about this exact topic. He explained that when we step into our truths, we will offend and scare those who are afraid to do the same. They will resent us because they see us manifesting their biggest fear, which is that total shedding of shame and that complete ownership of identity. They are still attached to apologizing for who they are, which makes our actions a violation of their worldview. They might even become hostile. But do not let this deter you. Why? Because for every person who resents your ability to speak out, there will be someone else who sees your empowerment as permission to do the same for themselves. They will see you and realize they don't have to apologize anymore. They will feel grateful and bonded to you because of the experience. And when they step into their truth? There will be more people who will see them and start doing the same. I still think about Dr Dream's talk all the time, because this is how we really change the world. We are all connected. You have no idea how stepping into your truth will create ripples, and enough ripples will create a tidal wave that will empower many other people to do the same. Empowerment spreads like wildfire, but it is up to you to light the match by simply refusing to apologize any longer for who you are. This is the single greatest form of resistance in a world of internet trolls and naysayers.

Tip 5: Practise Kindness (It's Free!)
It seems so simple, maybe too simple, but just being a good person will take you quite far in this life, especially when it comes to building relationships focused on growth, healing and positivity. If we plant the seeds for sex positive relationships in the garden of our lives, then kindness and compassion are the water and the sun that will help that garden bloom. You already know how to be a kind, loving person. Offer help to those in your life who need it, without an expectation of receiving anything in return. Be present and listen when people are speaking

their truths. Support those who are embracing their authentic selves, especially when others might mock them. Become an ally to those who are marginalized. Start a constructive dialogue with people who have different ideas from you. Pull your energy away from the low-hanging fruit of fighting with people on the internet. Maybe turn off social media altogether for a little while. Remember, energy flows where the attention goes. When you put your energy into being a loving, kind, supportive person, suddenly you will find that your relationships come to reflect these intentions and actions.

People often speak about dealing with "*energy vampires*" who will drain away all of your love and kindness and leave you dead inside. But we cannot avoid kindness and compassion out of fear of narcissists or toxic people. When that happens, we lose out on so many good things. If you are drawn to shower such energy vampires with all of your kindness (especially when you know better) then you are exhibiting a learned behaviour pattern which is keeping you from fully evolving into the person you were born to be.

In the same vein, we also know that we are not capable of kindness and compassion all the time, especially when we are living in a chaotic, ever shifting world that can cause us much stress and discomfort. Life is about balance, and being a good person is not about being positive all the time. It is about taking care of yourself so that you can hold space for others. When you are feeling like you cannot be kind to others, then it is time to disconnect, disengage and rekindle that kindness within yourself again. You are always allowed to feel and to work through your negative emotions, so long as you do not become trapped there in a toxic cycle of overthinking and self-hate. What do you do when your kindness has been drained? It is time to practise self-love, forgiveness, gratitude and flow, of course.

As with everything in this book, please remember that developing sex positive attitudes requires practice and hard work. I am right there with you, and I believe that you have more than enough power within yourself to build wonderful sex positive relationships. We never give up, we just keep learning, growing and moving forward!

NOTES

Introduction

1   C G Jung and Richard Francis Carrington Hull, *The Philosophical Tree* (London: Routledge and Kegan Paul, 1967), paragraph 335.

Chapter 1

2   Alia E Dastagir, "Gender Stereotypes Are Destroying Girls, and They're Killing Boys," *USA Today* (21 September 2017), www.usatoday.com/story/news/2017/09/21/gender-stereotypes-destroying-girls-and-theyre-killing-boys/68831 7001/

3   Robert W Blum, Kristin Mmari and Caroline Moreau, "It Begins at 10: How Gender Expectations Shape Early Adolescence around the World," *Journal of Adolescent Health*, 61 (2017), http://dx.doi.org/10.1016/j.jadohealth.2017.07.009

4   Ibid.

5   Shirley Donlon, "Kentucky Teen Says She Was Treated 'Like a Wh**e' and 'Humiliated' by Her High School After Being Sent Home for Wearing Short OVERALLS, Even Though They Didn't Violate the Dress Code," *Daily Mail UK* (23 April 2019), www.dailymail.co.uk/femail/article-6950681/Student-reveals-dress-coded-wearing-pair-overalls.html

6   Institute for Women's Policy Research, "Pay Equity and Discrimination," *Institute for Women's Policy Research* (2017), https://iwpr.org/issue/employment-education-economic-change/pay-equity-discrimination/

7   Kristen Bialik and Richard Fry, "Millennial Life: How Young Adulthood Today Compares with Prior Generations," *Pew Research Center* (2019), www.pewsocialtrends.org/essay/millennial-life-how-young-adulthood-today-compares-with-prior-generations/

8   American Society of Plastic Surgeons, "New Plastic Surgery Statistics Reveal Focus on Face and Fat," ASPS Press Release (1 March 2017), www.plasticsurgery.org/news/press-releases/new-plastic-surgery-statistics-reveal-focus-on-face-and-fat. At a show in Denver a few weeks ago, when I told the young woman next to me in the bathroom line what I did for a living, she immediately pulled down her pants and asked me if her labia was too large and if she should have surgery to get it reduced. I told her she was perfect the way she was.

9   United States Circumcision Incidence, *The Circumcision Reference Library,* www.cirp.org/library/statistics/USA/

10 Peter Moore, "Young Americans Less Supportive of Circumcision at Birth," *YouGov* (2015), https://today.yougov.com/topics/lifestyle/articles-reports/2015/02/03/younger-americans-circumcision

11 Harris O'Malley, "The Difference between Toxic Masculinity and Being a Man," *Good Men Project* (2016), https://goodmenproject.com/featured-content/the-difference-between-toxic-masculinity-and-being-a-man-dg/

12 "Parental Practices Analyzed: Exploring How Over 1,000 Approach Parenting," *Senior Living* (2019), www.seniorliving.org/research/parental-practices/

13 American Psychological Association, *Appropriate Affirmative Response to Sexual Orientation Distress and Change Efforts* (2009), www.apa.org/about/policy/sexual-orientation.pdf

14 Including the American Psychological Association, American Counselling Association, National Association of Social Workers, American Association of Paediatrics, American Psychiatric Association, American Association of School Counsellors, and more.

15 Tia Ghose, "Why Gay Conversion Therapy is Harmful," *Live Science* (10 April 2015), www.livescience.com/50453-why-gay-conversion-therapy-harmful.html

Chapter 2

16 The Gay and Lesbian Alliance Against Defamation Harris Poll, "Accelerating Acceptance," *GLAAD* (2017), www.glaad.org/files/aa/2017_GLAAD_Accelerating_Acceptance.pdf

17 Curtis Wong, "50 Percent of Millennials Believe Gender is a Spectrum, Fusion's Massive Millennial Poll Finds," *Huffington Post* (2015), www.huffpost.com/entry/fusion-millennial-poll-gender_n_6624200

18 Of millennials aged 18 and older, 25% knew someone who used a gender-neutral pronoun, compared with 35% of those aged 13–17. From "Gen-Z More Familiar With Gender Neutral Pronouns," *Pew Research Center* (2019), www.pewsocialtrends.org/2019/01/17/generation-z-looks-a-lot-like-millennials-on-key-social-and-political-issues/psdt_1-17-19_generations-02/

19 Other polls show 56% of Gen-Zs aged 13–20 knew someone who used a gender-neutral pronoun compared with 43% of millennials aged 28–34. From Shepherd Laughlin, "Gen-Z Goes Beyond Gender Binaries in Innovation Group Data," *J. Walter Thompson Intelligence* (2016), www.jwtintelligence.com/2016/03/gen-z-goes-beyond-gender-binaries-in-new-innovation-group-data/

20 One-third of Gen-Z respondents and younger millennials said that gender did not define them as a person, compared with 23% of older millennials aged 28–34, and 44% of Gen-Z said they would only buy clothes designed for their own gender compared with 54% of millennials. From Laughlin.

21 Lauren Friendman, "Millennials and Gender Fluidity – What Smart Brands Are Doing and Why," *Forbes* (2017), www.forbes.com/sites/laurenfriedman/2017/11/28/

millennials-and-gender-fluidity-what-smart-brands-are-doing-and-why/#7a13e7635436

22 About 1 in 2,000 children are born with chromosomes other than XX or XY leading to ambiguous genitalia. Until recently in the US, the doctor would make the decision to assign the sex to either male or female, which often resulted in multiple surgeries beginning at birth and causing terrible trauma to the individual and their families. Nowadays, more and more doctors are opting out of assigning sex, and allowing the family and child to decide at a more appropriate time.

23 A wealth of useful terms when it comes to the psychology of gender can be found here: "Definitions Related to Sexual Orientation and Gender Diversity," *American Psychological Association,* www.apa.org/pi/lgbt/resources/sexuality-definit ions.pdf

24 Around 0.7% of the total population of adults aged 18–24 identifies as transgender. All of the statistics are presented in A Flores, Jody Herman, Gary Gates and Taylor Brown, "How Many Adults Identify as Transgender in the United States?" *Williams Institute* (2016), http://williamsinstitute. law.ucla.edu/wp-content/uploads/How-Many-Adults-Identify-as-Transgender-in-the-United-States.pdf

25 Aruna Saraswat, Jamie Weinand and Joshua Safer, "Evidence Supporting the Biologic Nature of Gender Identity," *Endocrine Practice,* 21 (2015), 199–204, http://dx.doi.org/ 10.4158/ep14351.ra. Compare millennials' rate of 15% to only 7% of those aged 35–54 who ever felt that their gender identity does not match their sex at birth. From *YouGov,* 2015.

26 Ruby Rose as interviewed in *Elle Magazine* (15 June 2015), www.elle.com/culture/movies-tv/a28865/ruby-rose-oitnb/?src=spr_FBPAGE

27 Jessica Bennet, "She? Ze? They? What's in a Gender Pronoun?" *New York Times* (30 January 2016), www.

nytimes.com/2016/01/31/fashion/pronoun-confusion-sexual-fluidity.html

28 Centazi Nicholas Metcalf gave a Ted Talk on "Why We Need Gender Fluidity," *TED* (2015), www.youtube.com/watch?v=ICWB8pfGBvc

29 The founder of modern sex research, A C Kinsey, co-wrote with B Pomeroy and C E Martin, *Sexual Behavior in the Human Male* (Philadelphia: W B Saunders, 1948) and with B Pomeroy, C E Martin and P Gebhard, *Sexual Behavior in the Human Female* (Philadelphia: W B Saunders, 1953).

30 Kristin A Broussard and Ruth H Warner, "Gender Nonconformity Is Perceived Differently for Cisgender and Transgender Targets," *Sex Roles*, 80 (2018), 409–28, http://dx.doi.org/10.1007/s11199-018-0947-z

31 K Blair, "What Exactly Do Transgender People Threaten?" *Psychology Today* (24 September 2018), www.psychologytoday.com/us/blog/inclusive-insight/201809/what-precisely-do-transgender-people-threaten

32 An excellent elaboration of the discussion on transgender myths can be found here: G. Lopez, "Transgender People: 10 Common Myths," *Vox* (14 November 2018), www.vox.com/identities/2016/5/13/17938090/transgender-people-tricks-confused

33 D Trotta, "Exclusive: Women, Young People More Open on Transgender Issue in United States," *Reuters/Ipsos Poll* (2016), www.reuters.com/article/us-usa-lgbt-poll-idUSKCN0XI11M

34 Saraswat, Weinand and Safer.

35 Transequality.org: https://transequality.org/sites/default/files/docs/resources/Trans-People-Bathroom-Access-July-2016.pdf. USA Today / Rock the Vote Poll in 2016: www.usatoday.com/story/news/politics/onpolitics/2016/08/15/millennials-consensus-transgender-bathroom-use/8875 1928/

36 Vital information for those looking to become better transgender allies: "Tips for Allies of Transgender People," *GLAAD* (June 2018), www.glaad.org/transgender/allies

Chapter 3

37 A Yaroshenko, "What Is the SexTech Industry & How Is It Worth $30.6bn?" *Global Dating Insights* (23 June 2016), https://globaldatinginsights.com/2016/06/23/what-is-sextech-and-how-is-the-industry-worth-30-6-billion-developing/

38 C Gallop, "What is Sextech and Why Is Everyone Ignoring It?" *Hot Topics* (2017), www.hottopics.ht/14192/what-is-sextech-and-why-is-everyone-ignoring-it/

39 R Dawson and J Owsianik, "The Future of Sex Report" (2016), https://futureofsex.net/future-of-sex-report/

40 Sources vary, such as M Castleman, "Dueling Statistics: How Much of the Internet Is Porn?" *Psychology Today* (3 November 2016), www.psychologytoday.com/blog/all-about-sex/201611/dueling-statistics-how-much-the-internet-is-porn

41 While the Barna Group's 2014 *Proven Men Porn Survey* showed that 79% of American men and 76% of American women watched porn monthly, www.provenmen.org/2014PornSurvey/, porn watchdogs Covenant Eyes found in 2015 that 63% of millennial-aged men and 21% of women watched porn several times per week, www.covenanteyes.com/pornstats. Another study of 1,200 people in romantic relationships found that 44% of couples even reported watching porn together: Amanda M Maddox, Galena K Rhoades and Howard J Markman, "Viewing Sexually-Explicit Materials Alone or Together: Associations with Relationship Quality," *Archives of Sexual Behavior*, 40 (2009), 441–48, http://dx.doi.org/10.1007/s10508-009-9585-4

42 Pornhub, *Year in Review* (2018), www.pornhub.com/insights/2016-year-in-review. In this discussion we focus upon Pornhub because of the transparency and accessibility of their data, but please keep in mind this is only one of many porn sites on the web!

43 S Vannier, A Currie and L O'Sullivan, "Schoolgirls and Soccer Moms: A Content Analysis of Free 'Teen' and 'MILF' Online Pornography," *Journal of Sex Research*, 51.3 (2013), 253–64, www.tandfonline.com/doi/abs/10.1080/00224499.2013.829795

44 J Lehmiller, "Why Do Guys Like MILFs?" *Playboy Magazine* (2014), www.lehmiller.com/blog/2014/8/25/the-appeal-of-the-milf

45 This was absolutely the case for me and lesbian scissoring, and I wonder how many other women are searching for it just to see how it works! I had tried it a couple of times and genuinely could not figure out how to orgasm. For a while, I was convinced that scissoring was a made-up porn thing, but I watched enough of it and eventually did figure it out. It is all about the angles and the clit rubbing, in case you were wondering.

46 J Williams, "Quarter of Young Straight Women Have Had Lesbian Sex, While Half Believe Gender Is Fluid," *Pink News* (11 May 2016), www.pinknews.co.uk/2016/05/11/quarter-of-straight-women-have-had-lesbian-sex-while-half-believe-gender-is-fluid/

47 D Ley, Nicole Prause and Peter Finn, "The Emperor Has No Clothes: A Review of the 'Pornography Addiction' Model," *Current Sexual Health Reports*, 6 (2014), 94–105, https://link.springer.com/article/10.1007/s11930-014-0016-8

48 Simone Kühn and Jürgen Gallinat, "Brain Structure and Functional Connectivity Associated with Pornography Consumption," *JAMA Psychiatry*, 71 (2014), 827, http://dx.doi.org/10.1001/jamapsychiatry.2014.93

49 V Voon and others, "Neural Correlates of Sexual Cue Reactivity in Individuals With and Without Compulsive

Sexual Behaviours," *PLOS One*, 9 (2014), https://doi.org/10.1371/journal.pone.0102419

50 American Psychiatric Association, *Diagnostic Statistical Manual of Psychology* (DSM-V), Fifth Edition (Washington, DC: American Psychiatric Association Publishing, 2013), p. 481.

51 Matthias Brand and others, "Integrating Psychological and Neurobiological Considerations Regarding the Development and Maintenance of Specific Internet-Use Disorders: An Interaction of Person-Affect-Cognition-Execution (I-PACE) Model," *Neuroscience & Biobehavioral Reviews*, 71 (2016), 252–66, http://dx.doi.org/10.1016/j.neubiorev.2016.08.033

52 N Bahadur, "People Who Watch More Porn Have More Sex, Survey Finds", *Huffington Post* (February 2014), www.huffingtonpost.com/2014/02/11/porn-survey-have-more-sex_n_4746416.html

53 D Gaudiosi, "How Virtual Reality Could Improve Your Sex Life", *Fortune Magazine* (28 January 2016), http://fortune.com/2016/01/28/virtual-reality-sex-life/

54 C Nash, "EXCLUSIVE: Futurologist Dr Ian Pearson on Sex With Robots, Contact Lens VR, and More," *Brietbart Tech* (5 July 2016), www.breitbart.com/tech/2016/07/05/exclusive-people-will-emotional-sex-robots-2030-according-futurologist-dr-ian-pearson

55 Dawson and Owsianik.

56 R Waugh, "Male Sex Robots with Unstoppable Bionic Penises Are Coming This Year," *Metro UK* (8 January 2018), http://metro.co.uk/2018/01/08/male-sex-robots-unstoppable-bionic-penises-coming-year-7213306/

57 B Kerr, "Future Sex: How Close Are Robotic Love Dolls?" *Rolling Stone Magazine* (30 August 2017), www.rollingstone.com/culture/features/future-of-sex-how-close-are-robotic-love-dolls-w500191

58 Coined in 1970 by Japanese robotics professor Masahiro Miro, the *uncanny valley* hypothesis predicts that there is

a positive relationship between a robot's human likeness and our affinity to it, but only up to a certain point. The point occurs when robots appear *almost* exactly human, causing people to experience feelings of revulsion (aka that creepy, unsettling feeling). Theoretically, once the robot appears perfectly lifelike (a feat that engineers have yet to achieve) human reactions to them will become positive once again.

59 B Pemberton, "Brothel Shells Out £6,000 for its Second Sex Doll … After Their First Became MORE Popular with Customers Than Real Women," *Sun* (22 August 2017), www.thesun.co.uk/living/4296637/brothel-shells-second-sex-doll-first-more-popular-with-customers-than-real-women/

60 Ian Pearson, "The Future of Sex Report: The Rise of Robosexuals," *Bondara* (2015), http://graphics.bondara.com/Future_sex_report.pdf

61 Aaron Smith and Janna Anderson, "AI, Robotiocs, and the Future of Jobs," *Pew Research Center* (2014), www.pewinternet.org/2014/08/06/future-of-jobs/

62 J Szczuka and N Krämer, "Not Only the Lonely – How Men Explicitly and Implicitly Evaluate the Attractiveness of Sex Robots in Comparison to the Attractiveness of Women, and Personal Characteristics Influencing This Evaluation," *Multimodal Technologies and Interaction*, 1.1, 3 (2017), https://doi.org/10.3390/mti1010003

63 Dawson and Owsianik.

64 Jack Callil, "The Surprisingly Sensitive World of Men Who Own Sex Dolls," *Vice* (16 February 2015), www.Vice.com/en_us/article/dpwnwy/the-surprisingly-sensitive-world-of-men-who-own-sex-dolls

65 David Levy, *Love and Sex with Robots: The Evolution of Human-Robot Relationships* (New York: Harper Perennial, 2009).

66 Neil Mcarthur and Markie L C Twist, "The Rise of Digisexuality: Therapeutic Challenges and Possibilities,"

Journal of Sexual and Relationship Therapy, 32.3–4 (2017), Special Issue on Sex and Technology, 334–44.

67 C Nash, "Chinese Chatbot Has Been Told 'I Love You' Nearly 20 Million Times," *Brietbart Tech* (9 March 2017), www.breitbart.com/tech/2017/03/09/chinese-chatbot-told-love-nearly-20-million-times/

68 Dawson and Owsianik.

69 Nash, "EXCLUSIVE: Futurologist Dr. Ian Pearson On Sex With Robots."

70 Dawson and Owsianik.

71 Tom Woodley, "Transhumanism and the Future of Sex," *Future of Sex* (28 September 2017), https://futureofsex.net/augmentation/transhumanism-future-sex/

Chapter 4

72 Dana Macy, "2016 Yoga in America Study," *Yoga Journal* and *Yoga Alliance* (13 January 2016), http://media.yogajournal.com/wp-content/uploads/2016YIAS-Release-Final.pdf

73 Vikas Dhikav and others, "Yoga in Male Sexual Functioning: A Noncompararive Pilot Study," *Journal of Sexual Medicine*, 7.10 (2010), 3560-66, www.ncbi.nlm.nih.gov/pubmed/2064 6186 and Vikas Dhikav and others, "Yoga in Female Sexual Functions," *Journal of Sexual Medicine*, 7.2 (2010), 964–70, www.ncbi.nlm.nih.gov/pubmed/19912493

74 Thomas Currant and Andrew Hill, "Perfectionism Is Increasing Over Time: A Meta-Analysis of Birth Cohort Differences from 1989 to 2016," *Psychological Bulletin*, 145 (2019), 410–29, http://dx.doi.org/10.1037/bul0000138

75 Louise Hay, *You Can Heal Your Life* (London: Hay House Publishers, 1984).

76 Becca Alper, "Millennials Are Less Religious Than Older Americans, but Just as Spiritual," *Pew Research Center* (23 November 2015), www.pewresearch.org/fact-tank/2015/11/23/millennials-are-less-religious-than-older-americans-but-just-as-spiritual/ and Pew Research Center

Forum, "When Americans Say They Believe in God, What Do They Mean?" *Pew Research Center* (25 April 2018), www.pewforum.org/2018/04/25/when-americans-say-they-believe-in-god-what-do-they-mean/

77 Katie Richards, "Want to Win Over Millennials? Vice's New Study Says Brands Should Get Spiritual," *AdWeek* (19 June 2018), www.adweek.com/brand-marketing/want-to-win-over-millennials-and-gen-z-vices-new-study-says-brands-should-get-spiritual/

78 Karl Paul, "Why Millennials Are Ditching Religion for Witchcraft and Astrology," *Market Watch* (31 October 2018), www.marketwatch.com/story/why-millen nials-are-ditching-religion-for-witchcraft-and-astrology-2017-10-20

79 Brooks Hays, "Majority of Young Adults Think Astrology Is a Science," *UPI* (12 February 2014), www.upi.com/Science_News/2014/02/11/Majority-of-young-adults-think-astrology-is-a-science/5201392135954/

80 Kenzie Bryant, "Goop's Infamous Yoni Egg Cost the Company $145,000," *Vanity Fair* (5 September 2018), www.vanityfair.com/style/2018/09/gwyneth-paltrow-goop-jade-egg-lawsuit-settlement

81 Ellen Huet, "The Dark Side of the Orgasmic Meditation Company," *Bloomberg Business Week* (18 June 2018), www.bloomberg.com/news/features/2018-06-18/the-dark-side-of-onetaste-the-orgasmic-meditation-company

82 Chris Tognnotti, "Bikram Choudry's Accusers Reveal Harrowing Details of Their Allegations in ESPN's '30 for 30' Podcast," *Bustle* (26 May 2018), www.bustle.com/p/bikram-choudhurys-accusers-reveal-harrowing-details-of-their-allegations-in-espns-30-for-30-podcast-9215715

83 Michael C Mithoefer and others, "The Safety and Efficacy of ±3,4-Methylenedioxymethamphetamine-Assisted Psychotherapy in Subjects with Chronic, Treatment-Resistant Posttraumatic Stress Disorder: The First Randomized Controlled Pilot Study," *Journal of Psychopharmacology*, 25.4 (2011), 439–52, https://doi.org/10.1177/0269881110378371

84 Katie Anderson, "The MDMA Bubble: A Clean Slate of Communication for Couples," (Psychology Department, London Southbank University, 2016), www.essd-research.eu/ documents/ESSD%20presentations%202016/Katie%20 Anderson.pdf. For more information on MDMA, see *The Vaults of Erowid*, www.erowid.org/chemicals/mdma/ mdma.shtml

85 Cat McShane, "Refinery29: The Couples That Take MDMA Stay Together," *Multidisciplinary Association For Psychedelic Studies* (25 April 2017), https://maps.org/news/ media/6659-refinery29-the-couples-that-take-mdma-to-stay-together-2

86 See the interview with Dee Dee Goldpaugh in Michael Aaron, "Open Your Mind: Merging Psychedelic Therapy with Sex Therapy," *Psychology Today* (24 October 2017), www.psychologytoday.com/intl/blog/standard-deviations/ 201710/open-your-mind-merging-psychedelic-therapy-sex-therapy?amp=&fbclid=IwAR1WCA0wOI3xU84soeJ2 uRA_UIkycqEYxdpM6WNccOTMqtKxytTVYhFwtlA

87 Simon Romero, "In Brazil, Some Inmates Get Therapy with Hallucinogenic Tea," *New York Times* (28 March 2015), www.nytimes.com/2015/03/29/world/americas/a-hallucinogenic-tea-time-for-some-brazilian-prisoners. html. Just to clarify, I am not advocating for the self-administered use of psychedelics for any purposes, including sex therapy. Please wait a few years and you will be able to do this legally, in the safety of a professional's office using lab grade clean medicine, rather than the potentially adulterated, illegal garbage out on the street! In the era of prohibition, ingesting any psychedelic substance can constitute a significant risk and should not be undertaken without the assistance of a physician or mental health care professional in an approved, legal setting.

88 Osho, *Sex Matters* (New York: St Martins Griffin, 2003) p. 20.

89 Anaiya Sophia, *Sacred Sexual Union: The Alchemy of Love, Power, and Wisdom* (Rochester, VT: Destiny Books, 2013), p. 3.

90 Sunyata Saraswati and Bodhi Avinasha, *Jewel in the Lotus: The Tantric Path to Higher Consciousness: A Complete and Systematic Course in Tantric Kriya Yoga* (Valley Village, CA: Ipsalu Tantra, 2002), p. 21.

91 Anaiya Sophia explains in *Sacred Sexual Union*, p. 3.

92 Jolan Chang, *The Tao of Love: The Ancient Chinese Way to Ecstasy* (London: Wildwood House, 1977).

93 Masters and Johnson developed the *Squeeze Technique* in 1970 to help delay male ejaculation, which involves pressing and squeezing the glans (or head) of the penis during intercourse to cease building stimulation. Because this interrupts lovemaking, other sexologists have suggested squeezing at the base of the penis (known as a basilar squeeze, where the penis meets the scrotum) for 4–8 seconds during intercourse. For a brief summary of these techniques, see Ramesh Mahashewari, "Squeeze It the Right Way," *Practo* (22 July 2016), www.practo.com/healthfeed/squeeze-it-the-right-way-22885/post

94 Hsi Lai, *The Sexual Teachings of the White Tigress: Secrets of the Female Taoist Masters* (Rochester, VT: Destiny Books, 2001).

95 Ibid., p. 13.

96 Ibid., p. 62.

97 Gordon Gallup, Rebecca L Burch and Steven M Platek, "Does Semen Have Antidepressant Properties?" *Archives of Sexual Behavior*, 31.3 (2002), 289–93, https://link.springer.com/article/10.1023/A:1015257004839

98 Saraswati and Avinasha.

99 Amara Charles, *The Sexual Teachings of Quodoushka* (Rochester, VT: Destiny Books, 2011). pp. 111–16.

100 Ibid., p. 216.

101 Lisa Chase Patterson quoted in Milica Vladova, "The Importance of Our Sexual Partners," *Mind Body and*

Spirit WellBeing (7 November 2014), http://mindbody andspiritwellbeing.com/importance-sexual-partners/

Chapter 5

102 Emily Nagoski, *Come As You Are: The Surprising New Science That Will Transform Your Sex Life* (New York: Simon & Schuster, 2015).

103 *Telegraph*, "Want a Good Night's Sleep? Have Sex Say Doctors!" (26 July 2009), www.telegraph.co.uk/news/ health/5911373/Want-a-good-nights-sleep-Have-sex-say-doctors.html

104 N Magon and S Kalra, "The Orgasmic History of Oxytocin: Love, Lust and Labor," *Indian Journal of Endocrinology and Metabolism*, 15 Suppl 3 (September 2011), S156–61, www.ncbi.nlm.nih.gov/pmc/articles/PMC3183515/

105 Susan Hall and others, "Sexual Activity, Erectile Dysfunction and Incident Cardiovascular Events," *American Journal of Cardiology*, 105.2 (2010), 192–97, https://doi.org/10.1016/j.amjcard.2009.08.671

106 J R Rider and others, "Ejaculation Frequency and Risk of Prostate Cancer: Updated Results with an Additional Decade of Follow-up," *European Urology*, 70.6 (2016), 974–82, www.ncbi.nlm.nih.gov/pubmed/?term=10.1016/j.eururo.2016.03.027

107 Barry Komisaruk, Carlos Beyer-Flores and Beverly Whipple, *The Science of Orgasm* (Baltimore, MD: Johns Hopkins University Press, 2006). When I read a journal article on this topic that specifically mentioned female self-stimulation (masturbation) and pain regulation, I began masturbating regularly during my painful periods as a way to receive pain relief, and it did help a little bit!

108 Anke Hambach and others, "The Impact of Sexual Activity on Idiopathic Headaches: An Observational Study," *Cephalalgia: An International Journal of Headache*, 33.6 (2013), 384–89, www.ncbi.nlm.nih.gov/pubmed/23430983

109 Carol Rinkleib Ellison, *Women's Sexualities* (Read File Publishing, USA, 2006).

110 Erica R Glasper and Elizabeth Gould, "Sexual Experience Restores Age-Related Decline in Adult Neurogenesis and Hippocampal Function," *Hippocampus*, 23.4 (2013), 303–12, www.ncbi.nlm.nih.gov/pubmed/23460298

111 Jean M Twenge, Ryne A Sherman and Brooke E Wells, "Sexual Inactivity During Young Adulthood Is More Common Among U.S. Millennials and IGen: Age, Period, and Cohort Effects on Having No Sexual Partners After Age 18," *Archives of Sexual Behavior*, 46.2 (2017), 433–40, www.ncbi.nlm.nih.gov/pubmed/27480753

112 Ibid.

113 SKYN Condoms by Lifestyles, "2017 SKYN® Condoms Millennial Sex Survey Reveals Nearly 50% of Respondents Sext at Least Once Per Week," *PRNewsWire* (6 February 2017), www.prnewswire.com/news-releases/2017-skyn-condoms-millennial-sex-survey-reveals-nearly-50-of-respondents-sext-at-least-once-a-week-300401985.html

114 TENGA, "United States of Masturbation," (2016), www.tenga-global.com/campaign/UnitedStatesof Masturbation/

115 "Millennials Are Ruining America's Sex Life" (7 March 2017), www.ibtimes.co.uk/millennials-are-ruining-americas-sex-life-1610203; "Millennials Are Killing Sex, Beer, and Just About Everything Else Apparently" (2017), https://thetab.com/us/temple/2017/07/28/millennials-are-killing-sex-beer-and-just-about-everything-else-apparently-11632; "Millennial Sex Sucks" (19 May 2017), https://nypost.com/2017/05/19/why-millennial-sex-sucks/

116 Centers for Disease Control and Prevention, "Sexual Behavior, Sexual Attraction and Sexual Identity in the United States: Data from the 2006–2008 National Survey of Family Growth," *National Health Statistic Reports*, 36 (2011), www.cdc.gov/nchs/data/nhsr/nhsr036.pdf

117 Max Borges Agency, "How America's Largest Living Generation Shops Amazon," (2017), www.max

borgesagency.com/how-americas-largest-living-generation-shops-amazon/

118 Nagoski, p. 271.

119 Ibid., p. 66.

120 Komisaruk, Beyer-Flores and Whipple.

121 Nagoski, p. 283.

122 Charles, p. 202.

123 Ibid., p. 203.

124 Nagoski, p. 280.

125 Charles, p. 202.

126 Nagoski, p. 274.

127 One of the other common misconceptions is that men should always be ready for sex, and if they are not hard when it comes time, then their partner should take this personally as a sign that their man isn't interested or turned on by them. We need to stop putting this pressure on people, because as we will see in a little bit, the genitals don't always do what the mind tells them to do!

128 Nagoski, p. 69.

129 Ibid., p. 244.

130 Zara Stone, "Why the Smart Sex Toy Revolution Will Change Your Life," *Ackerman Forbes* (20 July 2017), www.forbes.com/sites/zarastone/2017/07/20/why-the-smart-sex-toy-revolution-will-change-your-life/#6337dffd38d6?

131 Alberto Rubio-Casillas and Emmanuele A Jannini, "New Insights from One Case of Female Ejaculation," *Journal of Sexual Medicine*, 8.12 (2011), 3500–4, www.ncbi.nlm.nih.gov/pubmed/21995650

132 Samuel Salama and others, "Nature and Origin of 'Squirting' in Female Sexuality," *Journal of Sexual Medicine*, 70.6 (2014), 974–82, https://onlinelibrary.wiley.com/doi/abs/10.1111/jsm.12799

133 Dawson and Owsianik, p. 21.

134 Jason Silva, "The Future of Sex," *YouTube* (2015), www.youtube.com/watch?v=9RTVrQARGhM

135 Dawson and Owsianik, p. 22.

136 Komisaruk, Beyer-Flores and Whipple.
137 Allura Joy, "How to Experience a Mindgasm that Rivals Your Most Intense Orgasm," *Your Tango* (21 July 2016), www.yourtango.com/experts/allura-joy/how-experience-mindgasm
138 Eyal Matsliah, *Orgasm Unleashed: Your Guide to Pleasure, Healing and Power* (Intimate Power, Australia, 2015).

Chapter 6

139 Bruce H Lipton, *The Biology of Belief: Unleashing the Power of Consciousness, Matter and Miracles* (Carlsbad, CA: Hay House, Inc., 2016).
140 I recommend PSYCH-K created by Rob Williams and Bruce Lipton. PSYCH-K offers a unique blend of various tools for changing subconscious beliefs, some contemporary and some ancient, derived from modern-day neuroscience research, as well as ancient mind/body wisdom. It goes beyond the usual methods of affirmation, positive thinking and visualization to promote lasting change to self-limiting and self-sabotaging beliefs.
141 Danny Penman, *The Art of Breathing* (Newburyport, MA: Conari Press, 2018).
142 Vanessa Marin, "How to Start Healing after Sexual Trauma," *Life Hacker* (30 November 2017), https://lifehacker.com/how-to-start-healing-after-sexual-trauma-1820455497
143 Ibid.
144 Julia Cameron, *The Artist's Way* (London: Pan Books, 1995).
145 L L Touissant, G S Shields and G M Slavich, "Forgiveness, Stress, and Health: A 5-Week Dynamic Parallel Process Study," *Annals of Behavioral Medicine*, 50.5 (2016), 727–35, www.ncbi.nlm.nih.gov/pubmed/27068160
146 Nathaniel Wade and others, "Efficacy of Psychotherapeutic Interventions to Promote Forgiveness: A Meta-Analysis," *Journal of Counseling and Clinical Psychology*, 82.1 (2014), 154–70, http://dx.doi.org/10.1037/a0035268

147 D Tibbits and others, "Hypertension Reduction through Forgiveness Training," *Journal of Pastoral Care and Counseling*, 60.1–2 (2016), 27–34, https://journals.sagepub.com/doi/abs/10.1177/154230500606000104

148 Frank D Fincham, Ross W May and Marcos A Sanchez-Gonzalez, "Forgiveness and Cardiovascular Functioning in Married Couples," *Couple and Family Psychology: Research and Practice*, 4.1 (2015), 39–48, www.fincham.info/papers/2015-forgive-cardio.pdf

149 Bob Enright quoted in Kristin Weir, "Forgiveness Can Improve Mental and Physical Health," *American Psychological Association Monitor on Psychology*, 48.1 (January 2017), www.apa.org/monitor/2017/01/ce-corner

150 Enright in Weir.

151 Wade and others.

152 Enright in Weir.

153 Mihaly Csikszentmihalyi, *Finding Flow in Everyday Life* (New York: Basic Books, 1998).

154 Mihaly Csikszentmihalyi interviewed by John Gerland, "Go with the Flow," *Wired Magazine* (1 September 1996), www.wired.com/1996/09/czik/

155 Gelman Gruber and Ranganath, "States of Curiosity Modulate Hippocampus-Dependent Learning via the Dopaminergic Circuit," *Neuron*, 84 (2014), 486–96, www.ncbi.nlm.nih.gov/pubmed/25284006

156 Carl Jung, *Letters* Vol. I, p. 33.

Chapter 7

157 *Oxford English Dictionary*, "Power Couple", www.lexico.com/en/definition/power_couple

158 Brittany Wong, "The 6 Relationship Problems Millennials Bring Up the Most in Therapy," *Huffington Post* (January 2018), www.huffpost.com/entry/millennials-most-common-relationship-problems_n_5a56581ce4b0a300f905371f

159 Gary Chapman, *The Five Love Languages* (Chicago, IL: Northfield Publishing, 1992).

160 Ibid.

161 Carmen Harra and Alexandra Harra, *The Karma Queens' Guide to Relationships: The Truth about Karma and Relationships* (New York: Penguin Group, 2015).

162 Ibid.

163 Robert J Sternberg, "A Triangle Theory of Love," *Psychological Review*, 93.2 (1986), 119–35, http://dx.doi.org/10.1037/0033-295X.93.2.119

164 R F Baumeister, "Passion, Intimacy, and Time: Passionate Love as a Function of Change in Intimacy," *Pers Soc Psychol Rev*, 3.1 (1999), 49–67, www.ncbi.nlm.nih.gov/pubmed/15647147

165 Elizabeth Gilbert quoted in Lisa Capretto, "Elizabeth Gilbert Explains What Everyone Gets Wrong about Soul Mates," *Huffington Post* (11 October 2014), www.huffpost.com/entry/elizabeth-gilbert-soul-mates_n_5961864?guccounter=1

166 Sophia, p. 13.

167 Ibid., p. 23.

Chapter 8

168 Karlyn Bowman, "Just How Many Spouses Cheat?" *Forbes Magazine* (19 June 2013), www.forbes.com/2009/06/28/sanford-ensign-affair-opinions-columnists-extramarital-sex.html#176b045edfdc

169 Eric Anderson, "Five Myths about Cheating," *Washington Post* (13 February 2012), www.washingtonpost.com/opinions/five-myths-about-cheating/2012/02/08/gIQANGdaBR_story.html?utm_term=.7856004bbc56

170 M W Wiederman and C Hurd, "Extradyadic Involvement during Dating," *Journal of Social and Personal Relationships*, 16.2 (1999), 265–74, https://doi.org/10.1177/0265407599162008

171 Jeanna Bryner, "Are Humans Meant to Be Monogamous?" *Live Science* (6 September 2012), www.livescience.com/32146-are-humans-meant-to-be-monogamous.html

172 Christopher Ryan and Cacilda Jethá, *Sex at Dawn: The Prehistoric Origins of Modern Sexuality* (Carlton: Scribe Publications, 2010).

173 Ibid., p. 11.

174 Ibid., p. 12.

175 Wendy Wang and Kim Parker, "Record Share of Americans Have Never Married," *Pew Research Center* (24 September 2014), www.pewsocialtrends.org/2014/09/24/record-share-of-americans-have-never-married/

176 Philip Cohen, "The Coming Divorce Decline," *SocArxivPapers* (14 September 2018), https://osf.io/preprints/socarxiv/h2sk6/

177 Jean M Twenge, *IGen: Why Todays Super-Connected Kids Are Growing Up Less Rebellious, More Tolerant, Less Happy – and Completely Unprepared for Adulthood: And What That Means for the Rest of Us* (New York: Atria Paperback, 2017).

178 Franklin Veaux and Eve Rickert, *More than Two: A Practical Guide to Ethical Polyamory* (Portland, OR: Thorntree Press, 2014), pp. 329–39, www.ncbi.nlm.nih.gov/pubmed/23541166

179 M L Haupert and others, "Prevalence of Experiences with Consensual Nonmonogamous Relationships: Findings from Two National Samples of Single Americans," *Journal of Sex & Marital Therapy*, 43 (2016), 424–40, http://dx.doi.org/10.1080/0092623x.2016.1178675

180 Terri Conley and others, "The Fewer the Merrier?: Assessing Stigma Surrounding Consensually Non-Monogamous Romantic Relationships," *Analyses of Social Issues and Public Policy*, 13 (2012), 1–30, http://dx.doi.org/10.1111/j.1530-2415.2012.01286.x

181 Justin Lehmiller, "Would Your Ideal Relationship Be Monogamous or Open? 1,000 Americans Weigh In," *Sex*

& *Psychology Blog* (31 October 2016), www.lehmiller.com/blog/2016/11/4/monogamous-and-open-relationships

182 Rhonda N Balzarini and others, "Perceptions of Primary and Secondary Relationships in Polyamory," *PLOS One*, 12 (2017), http://dx.doi.org/10.1371/journal.pone.0177841

183 Louisa Leontiades, "Relationship Fluidity Instead of Relationship Anarchy," (2016), http://louisaleontiades.com/relationship-fluidity-instead-of-relationship-anarchy/

184 M E Mitchell, K Bartholomew and R J Cobb, "Need Fulfillment in Polyamorous Relationships," *Journal of Sex Research*, 51.3 (2014), 329–39, https://doi.org/10.1080/00224499.2012.742998.

185 Chris Fleming, "Polyamorous," *YouTube* (2017), www.youtube.com/watch?v=DTsdKycVZZ4

186 "Compersion" gets bandied about all the time in CNM forums and communities, but you won't find it in the dictionary – unless you are looking in the *Urban Dictionary*. In terms of etymology, you can forget Greek, Latin or the Romance languages: A little bit of digging tells me that the term was actually invented sometime before 1985 by the members of the Kerista Commune in San Francisco, which lasted from mid 1970s to around 1991.

187 Veaux and Rickert, p. 458.

Chapter 9

188 Olivia Petter and Sarah Young, "Millennial Dating Trends 2019: All You Need to Know, from Ghosting to Bird Boxing," *Independent* (7 February 2019), https://independent.co.uk/life-style.love-sex/dating-trends-2109-terms-definitions-ghosting-orbiting-bird-boxing-millenial-a8767456.html

189 Phil Reed and others, "Differential Physiological Changes Following Internet Exposure in Higher and Lower Problematic Internet Users," *PLOS One*, 12 (2017), http://dx.doi.org/10.1371/journal.pone.0178480

190 International Center for Media and the Public Agenda (ICMPA) and the Salzburg Academy on Media and Global Change, "The World Unplugged Study" (2011), https://theworldunplugged.wordpress.com/

191 One meta-analysis found that 6% of the world's population, or 420 *million* people, are addicted to the Internet. China has even declared it a clinical disorder, but we remain more hesitant to do so in the West. See Cecilia Cheng and Angel Yee-Lam Li, "Internet Addiction Prevalence and Quality of (Real) Life: A Meta-Analysis of 31 Nations across Seven World Regions," *Cyberpsychology, Behavior, and Social Networking*, 17 (2014), 755–60, http://dx.doi.org/10.1089/cyber.2014.0317

192 Amanda Lenhart, "Social Media and Teen Friendships," *Pew Research Center* (6 August 2015), www.pewinternet.org/2015/08/06/chapter-4-social-media-and-friendships/

193 John Suler, "The Online Disinhibition Effect," *John Suler's Psychology of Cyberspace,* http://truecenterpublishing.com/psycyber/disinhibit.html

194 "Tinder Facts and Statistics," *Much Needed*, https://muchneeded.com/tinder-statistics/

195 ABODO Survey, "Swipe Right for Love? How 3,500 College Students Are Using Dating Apps" (28 March 2017), www.abodo.com/blog/swipe-right-love/

196 Jessica Strubel and Trent A. Petrie, "Love Me Tinder: Body Image and Psychosocial Functioning among Men and Women," *Body Image*, 21 (2017), 34–38, http://dx.doi.org/10.1016/j.bodyim.2017.02.006. A paper highlighting these findings was also presented at the American Psychological Association meeting in 2016.

197 Strubel and Petrie.

198 Ethan Kross and others, "Social Rejection Shares Somatosensory Representations with Physical Pain," *Proceedings of the National Academy of the Sciences of the United States of America*, 108.15 (2011), 6270–75, https://doi.org/10.1073/pnas.1102693108

199 Ernst Olav Botnen and others, "Individual Differences in Sociosexuality Predict Picture-Based Mobile Dating App Use," *Personality and Individual Differences*, 131 (2018), 67–73, http://dx.doi.org/10.1016/j.paid.2018.04.021

200 Lenhart.

201 CDC suicide rate review, Oren Miron and others, "Suicide Rates Among Adolescents and Young Adults in the United States, 2000–2017," *American Medical Association*, 321.23 (18 June 2019), 2362–64, https://jamanetwork.com/journals/jama/article-abstract/2735809

202 Lenhart.

203 J Holt-Lunstad and others, "Loneliness and Social Isolation as Risk Factors for Mortality: A Meta-analytic Review," *Perspectives on Psychological Science*, 10.2 (11 March 2015), 227–37, https://doi.org/10.1177/1745691614568352

RECOMMENDED READING

Introduction
Resources for the #MeToo movement: https://metoomvmt.org/ resources/

Support for women with uterine fibroids: www.nichd.nih.gov/ health/topics/uterine/conditioninfo/treatments/support

"Teaching Consent": www.teachconsent.org/

The Tryst Network sex positive resource: http://trystnetwork. org/about/

"Understanding Consent": www.rainn.org/understanding-consent

Chapter 1
Cordelia Fine, *Delusions of Gender* (WW Norton & Company, 2011)

Peggy Orienstein, *Girls and Sex: Navigating the Complicated New Landscape* (Harper Books, 2017)

Gender Stereotype Resources
"Closing the Gender Pay Gap": www.learnhowtobecome .org/ career-resource-center/closing-the-gender-pay-gap/

Exercises for reducing gender stereotypes: www.tolerance.org/ classroom-resources/tolerance-lessons/what-are-gender-stereotypes

"Talking to Kids about Gender Stereotypes": http://media smarts.ca/tipsheet/talking-kids-about-gender-stereotypes-tip-sheet

End Victim Blaming/Slut Shaming Resources

Amber Rose Slut Walk: www.facebook.com/Slut Walk?/

"How to Avoid Victim Blaming" (Harvard Law School HALT): https://orgs.law.harvard.edu/halt/how-to-avoid-victim-blaming/

National Alliance to End Sexual Violence: www.endsexual violence.org/

Karley Sciotino, *Slutever: Dispatches from a Sexually Autonomous Woman in a Post-Shame World* (Grand Central Publishing, 2018)

Toxic Masculinity Resources

APA's first ever guidelines for practice with boys and men: www. apa.org/monitor/2019/01/ce-corner

Tips for addressing toxic masculinity in your community: https://goodmenproject.com/featured-content/how-you-can-reduce-toxic-masculinity-in-your-neighborhood-lbkr/

Jared Yates Sexton, *The Man They Wanted Me to Be: Toxic Masculinity and a Crisis of Our Own Making* (Counterpoint, 2019)

Body Positive Resources

Body acceptance worksheets: https://positivepsychology.com/ positive-body-image/

Megan Jayne Crabbe, *Body Positive Power: Because Life Is Already Happening and You Don't Need Flat Abs to Live It!* (Seal Press, 2018)

Dove Self-Esteem project: www.dove.com/us/en/dove-self-esteem-project/help-for-parents/media-and-celebrities.html

Jameela Jamil's "I Weigh": https://jameelajamil.co.uk/post/
171287759245/i-weigh

Sonya Renee Taylor, *This Body Is Not an Apology: The Radical
Power of Self Love* (Berrett-Koehler Publishers, 2018)

Chapter 2

Understanding Gender Identity

Creating gender inclusive environments: www.genderspectrum.
org/resources/

"How to Talk To Young Kids about Gender" (Talk With Your
Kids): www.talkwithyourkids.org/lets-talk-about/how-talk-
young-kids-about-gender.html

Micah Rajunov and A Scott Duane, *NonBinary: Memoirs of
Gender and Identity* (Columbia University Press, 2019)

"Trans + Gender Identity" (The Trevor Project): www.thetrevor
project.org/trvr_support_center/trans-gender-identity/

LGBTQI+ Support Resources

GLAAD transgender resources: www.glaad.org/trans gender/
resources

Human Rights Campaign: www.hrc.org

LGBTQI health and therapy resources: www.lgbthealth
education.org/lgbt-education/lgbt-health-resources/

Sexual orientation and gender identity resources for youth
(American Psychological Association): www.apa.org/pi/aids/
youth/sexual-orientation

Transgender Ally Resources

GLAAD: www.glaad.org/transgender/allies

Resources for people with transgender family members: www.
hrc.org/resources/resources-for-people-with-transgender-
family-members

Straight for Equality: www.straightforequality.org/transresources

TransEquality: https://transequality.org/issues/resources/supporting-the-transgender-people-in-your-life-a-guide-to-being-a-good-ally

Chapter 3

John Danaher and Neil McArthur, *Robot Sex: Social and Ethical Implications* (MIT Press, 2018)

Kate Devlin, *Turned On: Science, Sex and Robots* (Bloomsbury Sigma, 2018)

David Levy, *Love and Sex with Robots: The Evolution of Human–Robot Relationships* (Harper, 2007)

Emily Witt, *Future Sex* (Farrar, Strauss & Giroux, 2017)

Chapter 4

Modern Spirituality Resources

Sara Beak, *Redvelations: A Soul's Journey to Becoming Human* (Sounds True, 2018)

Gabrielle Bernstein, *The Universe Has Your Back* (Hay House, 2018)

Joe Dispenza, *Becoming Supernatural* (Hay House, 2018)

Louise Hay, *You Can Heal Your Life* (Hay House, 1984)

Ekhart Tolle, *The Power of Now* (Namaste Publishing, 2004)

Spiritual Sex Resources

Barbara Carrellas, *Urban Tantra, Second Edition: Sacred Sex for the 21st Century* (Ten Speed Press, 2017)

Jolan Chang, *The Tao of Love and Sex* (Penguin Compass, 1991)

Amara Charles, *The Sexual Practices of Quodoushka* (Destiny Books, 2011)

Mantak and Manewaan Chia, *Healing Love through the Tao* (Destiny Books, 2005)

Hsi Lai, *Sexual Teachings of the White Tigress* (Destiny Books, 2001)

Somraj Pokras and Jeffre Talltrees, *Tantric Pathways to Supernatural Sex* (Llewellyn, 2019)

Sunyata Saraswati and Bodhi Avinasha, *Jewel in the Lotus: The Tantric Path to Higher Consciousness* (Ipsalu Publishing, 2002)

Chapter 5

Ian Kerner, *She Comes First: The Thinking Man's Guide to Pleasuring a Woman* (William Morrow Paperbacks, 2009)

Barry Komisaruk, Carlos Beyer-Flores and Beverly Whipple, *The Science of Orgasm* (Johns Hopkins University Press, 2006)

Eyal Matsliah, *Orgasm Unleashed* (Intimate Power, 2015)

Emily Nagoski, *Come As You Are: The Suprising New Science That Will Transform Your Sex Life* (Simon & Schuster, 2015)

Xanet Pallet, *Living an Orgasmic Life: Heal Yourself and Awaken Your Pleasure* (Mango, 2018)

Andrea Pennington, *The Orgasm Prescription for Women* (Make Your Mark Global, 2016)

Tristan Taormino, *Fifty Shades of Kink: An Introduction to BDSM* (Cleis Press, 2014)

Chapter 6

Bruce Lipton, *The Biology of Belief: Unleashing the Power of Consciousness, Matter and Miracles* (Hay House, 2008)

Bruce Lipton's list of belief change and energy psychology modalities resources: www.brucelipton.com/other-resources

Dayna Mason and Jason Andrada, *Beyond #Metoo: Love Yourself and Take Back Your Life* (Create Space, 2017)

Meditation Resources

Free meditation resources: (podcasts, Spotify, YouTube, apps and more) https://choosemuse.com/blog/ultimate-list-of-free-meditation-resources/

Thich Naht Han, *Peace is Every Step: The Path of Mindfulness in Everyday Life* (Bantam, 1992)

Danny Penman, *The Art of Breathing* (Conari Press 2018)
Sonyal Rinpoche, *The Tibetan Book of Living and Dying 25th
    Anniversary Edition* (Harper San Francisco, 2012)
Transcendental meditation: www.tm.org
Vedic meditation: www.vedicpathmeditation.com

Forgiveness Resources
Mihaly Csikszentmihalyi, *Finding Flow in Everyday Life* (Basic
    Books, 1997)
Fred Luskin, *Forgive for Good* (Harper One, 2003)
Desmond Tutu and Mpho Tutu, *The Book of Forgiving: The Fourfold
    Path to Healing Ourselves and Our World* (Harper One, 2015)
Everett Worthington and Steven Sandage, *Forgiveness and
    Spirituality in Psychotherapy: A Relational Approach* (American
    Psychological Association, 2015)

Chapter 7
Gary Chapman, *The Five Love Languages: The Secret to Love that
    Lasts* (Northfield Publishing, 2015)
The Five Love Languages quizzes and profiles: www.5love
    languages.com/quizzes/
Carmen Harra and Alexandra Harra, *The Karma Queens' Guide
    to Relationships* (Tarcher Perigee, 2015)
Sue Johnson, *Hold Me Tight: Seven Conversations for a Lifetime
    of Love* (Little, Brown, Spark, 2008)
Amir Levine and Rachel Heller, *Attached: The New Science of
    Adult Attachment and How It Can Help You Find and Keep
    Love* (Tarcher Perigee, 2012)
Anaiya Sophia, *Sacred Sexual Union* (Destiny Books, 2013)

Chapter 8
Kitty Chambliss and Elizabeth Sheff, *Jealousy Survival Guide:
    How to Feel Safe, Happy and Secure in Open Relationships*
    (CreateSpace 2017)

Dossie Easton and Janet Hardy, *The Ethical Slut,* Third Edition (Ten Speed Press, 2017)

Kathy Labriola, *The Jealousy Workbook* (Greenery Press, 2013)

Christopher Ryan and Cacilda Jetha, *Sex at Dawn: How We Mate, Why We Stray, and What It Means for Modern Relationships* (Harper Perennial, 2011)

Tristan Taormino, *Opening Up: A Guide to Creating and Sustaining Open Relationships* (Cleis Press, 2008)

"Franklin Veaux's Map of Non-Monogamy" (Franklin Veaux, 2010–17): www.xeromag.com

Franklin Veaux and Eve Richart, *More than Two: A Practical Guide to Ethical Polyamory* (Thorntree Press, 2014). Also check out their polyamory resources: www.morethantwo.com/resources.html

Dedeker Winston, *The Smart Girl's Guide to Polyamory* (Skyhorse, 2017)

Chapter 9

Devorah Heitner, *Screenwise: Helping Kids Thrive and Survive in Their Digital World* (Routledge, 2018)

Sherry Turkle, *Alone Together: Why We Expect More from Technology and Less from Each Other* (Basic Books, Revised 2017)

Jean Twenge, *Generation Me: Why Today's Young Americans Are More Confident, Assertive, Entitled – and More Miserable Than Ever Before* (Atria Books, 2014)

Jean Twenge, *iGen: Why Today's Super-Connected Kids Are Growing Up Less Rebellious, More Tolerant, Less Happy – and Completely Unprepared for Adulthood – and What That Means for the Rest of Us* (Atria Books, 2017)